Breast Disease:
A Problem-Based Approach

Breast Disease:
A Problem-Based Approach

Edited by

J Michael Dixon BSc(Hons), MBChB, MD, FRCS, FRCS(Ed)
Honorary Senior Lecturer in Surgery, University of Edinburgh
and
Consultant Surgeon, Edinburgh Breast Unit, Western General Hospital, Edinburgh

Monica Morrow BS, MD, FACS
Professor of Surgery, Northwestern University Medical School
and
Director, Lynn Sage Comprehensive Breast Center, Northwestern Memorial Hospital, Chicago

W. B. SAUNDERS

London • Edinburgh • New York • Philadelphia • Sydney • Toronto

WB SAUNDERS
A Division of Harcourt Brace and Company Limited.

ISBN 0-7020-2325-6

First published 1999

British Library Cataloguing in Publication Data
A catalogue record for this book is available from the British Library

Library of Congress Cataloging in Publication Data
A catalog record for this book is available from the Library of Congress

Medical knowledge is constantly changing. As new information
becomes available, changes in treatment, procedures, equipment and
the use of drugs become necessary. The authors and Publishers have, as
far as is it is possible, taken care to ensure that the information given in
the text is accurate and up to date. However, readers are strongly
advised to confirm that the information, especially with regard to drug
usage, complies with latest legislation and standards of practice.

The
Publisher's
policy is to use
**paper manufactured
from sustainable forests**

Commissioning Editor: Rachel Stock
Project Editor: Rachel Robson
Project Supervisor: Mark Sanderson
Typeset by Paston PrePress Ltd, Beccles, Suffolk
Printed in Hong Kong

Contents

Contributors

Nigel J Bundred FRCS
Consultant Breast Surgeon
Reader in Surgical Oncology
Department of Surgery
University Hospital of South Manchester
Manchester
UK

J Michael Dixon BSc(Hons) MBChB MD
    FRCS FRCS(Ed)
Honorary Senior Lecturer
University of Edinburgh;
Consultant Surgeon
Edinburgh Breast Unit
Western General Hospital
Edinburgh
UK

William Gradishar MD
Associate Professor of Medicine
Director of Breast Medical Oncology
Northwestern University Medical School
Chicago, Illinois
USA

Robert CF Leonard BSc MB BS MD
    FRCP(Ed)
Senior Lecturer
University of Edinburgh;
Consultant Medical Oncologist
Edinburgh Breast Unit
Western General Hospital
Edinburgh
UK

Monica Morrow BS MD FACS
Professor of Surgery
Northwestern University Medical School;
Director
Lynn Sage Comprehensive Breast Center
Northwestern Memorial Hospital
Chicago, Illinois
USA

J Richard C Sainsbury MD FRCS
Consultant Surgeon
Huddersfield Royal Infirmary
Huddersfield
UK

Luz A Venta MD
Associate Professor of Radiology
Northwestern University Medical School
Chicago, Illinois
USA

James D Watson FRCS(Ed) FRCSG(Plast)
Consultant Plastic Surgeon
St John's Hospital at Howden
Livingston, West Lothian
UK

Yvonne T Wilson MBChB FRCS
    FRCS(Plast)
Consultant Plastic Surgeon
St John's Hospital at Howden
Livingston, West Lothian
UK

Acknowledgements

The original clinical photographs used in the text were taken by the Medical Photography Department at the Western General Hospital, Edinburgh. They were copied and prepared for final publication by Mr Dave Dirom of the Medical Illustration Department of the University of Edinburgh. All patients who had photographs taken gave permission for their use in medical textbooks and their help and co-operation is acknowledged. Mrs Carol Lindsay, Senior Radiographer in the X-Ray Department of the Edinburgh Breast Unit, provided assistance in identifying appropriate X-rays. Mr Basil Venizelos provided assistance in identifying appropriate references. The whole of the text was compiled and typed by Miss Monica McGill who also co-ordinated the illustrations. The successful completion of this project owes much to her patience and organizational skills. JMD acknowledges the support and understanding of Pam, Oliver and Jonathan, during the many evenings he spent editing and revising the text.

Introduction

There are numerous books covering all aspects of breast disease.
Why, therefore, is there any need for another book? The answer is
that there are problems with the textbooks that are currently
available. A woman does not present to hospital with a fibroadenoma,
she presents with a lump which then needs to be appropriately
assessed, investigated and a specific diagnosis obtained. It is this
patient-orientated approach that is missing from many texts which
provides the basis and *raison d'être* for this text. Through a series of
clinical scenarios we have tried to cover the major aspects of benign
and malignant disease. Our aim has been to provide a compact,
concise and practical textbook for doctors and ancillary staff involved
in the day-to-day management of patients with breast disease. Only
you as the reader can judge if we have succeeded.

J M Dixon
M Morrow

A 19-year-old with a skin lesion in the inframammary fold

N J Bundred

A 19-year-old girl presents because she has noticed a skin lesion in the inframammary fold of the breast (Figure 1.1). What is this lesion, what is the frequency of this condition and what treatment should be offered?

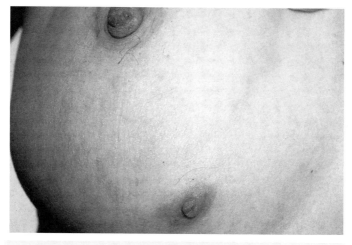

Fig. 1.1 Supernumerary/accessory nipple.

This is a supernumerary/accessory nipple. Accessory nipples are not usually associated with underlying breast tissue. Extra nipples are usually found along the embryonic milk line which runs from the axilla to the labia majora (Figure 1.2). They are most commonly seen below the breast, but also occur above the umbilicus or the abdomen or in the inframammary fold. The reported incidence varies between 0.2% and 2.5%. Accessory nipples are common and patients should be reassured they are of no importance. The nipple may occur alone or

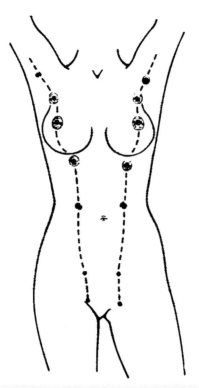

Fig. 1.2 Milk line.

have an associated areola. They are often mistaken for naevi. Usually no treatment is required for the condition. Occasionally the patient will request removal because she is embarrassed by it and, in such a case, it can be excised under local anaesthetic.

A 35-year-old with bilateral lumps in both axillae

N J Bundred

A 35-year-old presents with bilateral lumps in both axillae which she first noticed during her second pregnancy when they became tender and acutely enlarged. She has continued to complain of cyclical pain from the lumps and they enlarged again during a subsequent pregnancy and this led her to worry about the nature of these lumps (Figure 2.1). What is causing her symptoms and what management would you suggest?

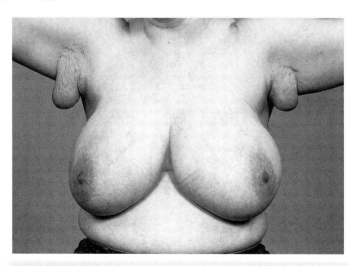

Fig. 2.1 Supernumerary/accessory breasts.

She presents with a classical history of accessory breast tissue which has enlarged during her second and third pregnancies, and bilateral accessory breasts are clearly visible in the clinical photograph. Although this breast tissue appears to have involuted after each pregnancy, she has continued to have breast pain and discomfort in the accessory tissue which is not unusual. Approximately 2% of women have accessory breasts with the majority not having associated nipples. Accessory breasts develop along the milk line and they are most commonly found in the lower axilla although they are sometimes seen below the breast (Figure 2.2). They are not seen as frequently in men. During pregnancy, hormonal stimulation causes enlargement. Many benign and malignant conditions have been described in accessory breasts, including ductal carcinoma *in situ* and invasive breast cancer.

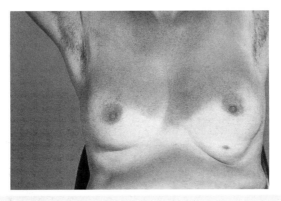

Fig. 2.2 Accessory breast just below normal left breast.

For those women in whom no more pregnancies are planned and the accessory breast is causing few symptoms, conservative management with reassurance is all that is necessary. If they are unsightly, both accessory breasts can be excised. It is important to take an ellipse of skin over the accessory breasts when performing surgery to ensure that the final skin wound is flat and cosmetically acceptable. Scars should remain posterior to the anterior axillary fold to ensure that they do not extend on to the anterior chest wall.

3 Marked breast asymmetry in a 19-year-old

Y T Wilson

A 19-year-old woman presents complaining of lack of development of the left breast. Her breasts started to develop at 11 years of age and, although this appeared to proceed normally on the right, there has been minimal development of the left breast. The other secondary sexual characteristics are normal and she has a regular menstrual cycle. She is shown in Figure 3.1. What is the diagnosis?

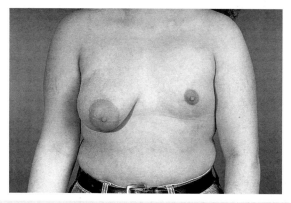

Fig. 3.1 Patient with hypoplasia of left breast.

She has unilateral hypoplasia.

What other features may be associated with unilateral breast hypoplasia?

There may be absence or deficiency of the sternocostal head of the ipsilateral pectoralis major muscle. When this occurs along with developmental abnormalities of the upper limb (specifically hypoplasia of the hand and forearm, short digits and syndactyly), it is known as

Poland's syndrome (Alfred Poland, 1841) (Figure 3.2). More severe cases may also exhibit a contracted anterior axillary fold, absence of pectoralis minor, hypoplasia of other chest wall muscles and deficiencies of the thoracic skeleton. Current theories suggest a vascular aetiology for Poland's syndrome and this is supported by the rare occurrence of Poland's syndrome in association with congenital palsy of the VIth and VIIth cranial nerves.

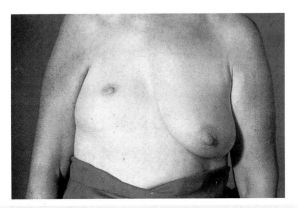

Fig. 3.2 Patient with Poland's syndrome.

Examination of the patient reveals no abnormalities of the upper limb, chest wall or musculature. She has a normal anterior axillary fold. What features of the right (unaffected) breast should be noted?

It is important to confirm that the supposedly well-developed breast is in fact normal. The size, shape, degree of ptosis and nipple position are all recorded, as the aim of surgery will be to achieve symmetry. The configuration of the larger breast is a major factor governing whether or not this will be possible.

The patient's right breast is of medium size with a minor degree of ptosis. She is satisfied with its appearance. The position of the right nipple is 21 cm from the sternal notch and the left nipple is at 19 cm. What surgical options would you consider to correct the asymmetry?

The most common approaches that should be considered are as follows:

1. Single stage augmentation of the hypoplastic breast
This is appropriate in certain cases and is most likely to be successful

where a degree of breast development has occurred on the hypoplastic side. In more severe cases of hypoplasia there is a relative deficiency of skin and it will be difficult to achieve symmetry with this technique. The resultant breast will tend to be small with the nipple in a high position.

2. Tissue expansion of the hypoplastic breast
This technique is usually employed when extra skin is required. Many shapes and sizes of expander are available and either a replaceable tissue expander or permanent expander prosthesis may be used. Once expansion is complete, the tissue expander is removed and replaced by a definitive prosthesis. The permanent expander prosthesis has a double lumen construction; the outer chamber is filled with silicone gel and the inner chamber is inflated to the required volume by injections of saline. The advantage of this device is that only the detachable injection port needs to be removed, so that the second surgical procedure is a relatively minor one. There are also newer product designs in which the injection port is incorporated into the main expander and therefore does not need to be removed.

3. Bilateral surgery
If the normally developed breast is large or ptotic, it is very difficult with either augmentation or tissue expansion of the hypoplastic breast to match it. In such cases, in addition to the surgery on the hypoplastic breast, the larger breast will require either a reduction or mastopexy procedure to achieve symmetry.

How would the management differ if there was an associated absence of the pectoralis major muscle?

In these cases with a more severe deformity, the latissimus dorsi muscle (providing it is uninvolved) gives the best reconstruction of the anterior chest wall. Transfer of the latissimus dorsi can be performed so as to produce an anterior axillary fold and provide adequate soft tissue cover for a tissue expander or prosthesis.

The patient undergoes insertion of a round 400 cc capacity Becker-type expander prosthesis in a left-sided submuscular pocket, through an inframammary incision. The dome-shaped injection port is placed in a subcutaneous pocket in the left axilla. Percutaneous injections of

saline are used to inflate the expander over a period of 4 months. What problems may be encountered during tissue expansion?

The early post-operative complications include haematoma, infection and delayed wound healing. Late infection is also seen and, if this occurs, the expander should be removed. A second attempt may be made several months later when the infection has settled. The most common problems with tissue expanders are of a mechanical nature: there may be failure of the device with leakage and deflation at any time during the expansion process. The injection port may be uncomfortable or become displaced, making inflation difficult. During expansion, irregularities known as 'knuckles' may develop on the surface of the expander and threaten the overlying skin. This is usually a direct result of poor surgical technique, where the expander is too large for the pocket that has been dissected. In such cases, any further inflation should proceed with caution to avoid necrosis of the overlying skin and exposure of the expander. Capsular contracture may occur around the expander with the formation of a dense layer of fibrous tissue around the expansion device. This can cause firmness and discomfort in the breast and may make further inflation of the expander difficult. Many patients undergoing expansion will develop striae of the breast and, if they are unsightly, it may be necessary to slow down the rate of expansion.

Patient compliance is occasionally a problem and the need to attend for multiple appointments must be discussed before embarking on such a course of treatment.

When the cumulative volume of saline injected into the expander totals 350 ml, the two breasts appear of similar size; however, the left breast is less ptotic than the right. How can the desired shape of the expanded breast be achieved and symmetry improved?

Many authors recommend a period of overinflation followed by later removal of some of the saline from the expander. This will produce a relative excess of skin and thus a certain degree of ptosis in the expanded breast. If the contralateral breast has only minor ptosis, this may be all that is required to achieve reasonable symmetry. If the normal breast is large or ptotic, even this manoeuvre will not produce symmetry and the remaining option is surgery to the larger breast once the expansion process is complete. In this patient, a further 150 ml of saline was injected and left for 3 months before it was removed. This produced a more naturally shaped breast, with a similar degree of ptosis to the right (unaffected) breast. No surgical procedure was therefore required to the left breast and the injection port was removed at 9 months when it was judged that no further adjustments to the breast volume would be required.

In the motivated patient with marked unilateral breast hypoplasia, tissue expansion is the technique most frequently used to increase breast volume. Patient management is largely dictated by the dimensions and characteristics of the well-developed breast and also whether or not they are willing to have any surgery to that breast. In most cases it should be possible to produce a reasonable degree of symmetry to the psychological and physical benefit of the patient (Figure 3.3).

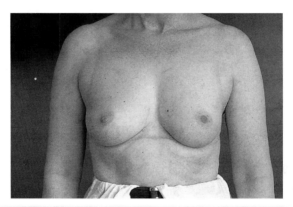

Fig. 3.3 Patient who had left breast hypoplasia treated by tissue expansion and replacement with a permanent prosthesis.

4 Large breasts in a 45-year-old

Mr J D Watson

A 45-year-old woman is referred by her general practitioner for consideration of breast reduction. She states that she has always had large breasts and now feels that this is responsible for her symptoms of back and neck ache (Figure 4.1). She is otherwise well and has had no previous significant illnesses. How would you manage her?

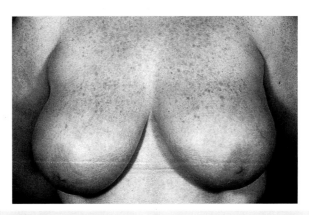

Fig. 4.1 Breast hyperplasia.

It is important to understand completely the woman's motivation for this type of surgery, which some might view as cosmetic. Breast reduction surgery is a significant procedure which can take as much as 3–4 hours to complete under general anaesthetic. It is associated with significant and permanent scarring, the quality of which cannot be predetermined.

The ideal candidate is one who has significantly large breasts. This can be gauged by asking their current bra size. Most would agree that a woman with a cup size of greater than DD is worthy of considering for reduction surgery. They should have physical symptoms related to the size of their breasts. Back and neck ache are the result of poor posture and the individual's attempt to conceal their large breasts. These symptoms will only respond to surgery if the woman corrects her poor posture. Grooving from the bra straps is a reliable sign of significantly large breasts (Figure 4.2). Submammary intertrigo should be inquired after. Women being considered for breast reduction should not be significantly overweight, i.e. their body mass index (BMI) should be less than 27. More obese individuals are prone to a higher risk of complications following surgery. Women with a BMI >27 should be encouraged to lose weight. In many, acceptance for breast reduction will prove to be the motivation for successful weight loss.

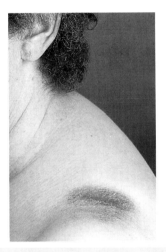

Fig. 4.2 Grooving from bra straps over shoulders in patient with breast hyperplasia.

The woman must realise that she is trading her large breasts for significant permanent scars and, in some, a degree of asymmetry. It is these two features which can reduce patient satisfaction if the sheer bulk of the breasts has not been the reason for seeking operation. In addition to the potential complications of any operation, i.e. bleeding, infection and those related to general anaesthesia, there are those which are specific to the operation of reduction mammaplasty. These are delayed healing, alteration in/loss of nipple sensation, possible inability to breast feed, nipple loss, fat necrosis and skin loss. Some form of complication has been reported in as many as 40% of patients.

When the reduction is particularly large, i.e. >1000 g, minor revisions to the scars may be required, especially in the intermammary area.

A 16-year-old girl who is completely healthy is referred because of breast hypertrophy ('virginal hypertrophy'). How would management of this girl differ?

In addition to discussing the range of potential problems outlined above, more emphasis needs to be placed on the permanency of scarring, alteration/loss of nipple sensation and difficulties with breast feeding. It is the need for a second and technically more demanding reduction operation. This may be avoided if primary surgery can be delayed until the patient is no longer a teenager (Figure 4.3).

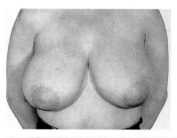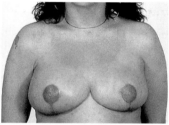

Fig. 4.3 Reduction surgery for breast hyperplasia. Patient before and after reduction surgery for hyperplasia.

Problem of small breasts in a 25-year-old

Y T Wilson

A 25-year-old woman presents requesting bilateral breast augmentation. She has always had very small breasts and wears a size 34A bra (Figure 5.1a). There has been no recent change in breast size or in her weight, which is within the normal range for her height. What reasons may she have for seeking surgery to increase the size of her breasts?

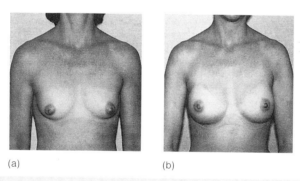

(a)   (b)

Fig. 5.1 Patient before (a) and after breast augmentation (b).

Most patients requesting breast enlargement are motivated by feelings of inadequacy and lack of self-esteem. This may have a detrimental effect on their interpersonal relationships. They also frequently describe a lack of self-confidence which affects their social interactions and sometimes their performance at work. It is important to discuss why she wishes to change her body image and to uncover at this stage any psychological or psychiatric problems. On occasion there may be a serious underlying psychological disorder which should be fully explored before any surgery is undertaken. Such patients are not good candidates for surgery.

What aspects of the medical history are relevant?

Specific enquiry should be made concerning any personal or family history of benign breast disease or breast cancer. A history of past pregnancies and any significant changes in the breasts at that time should be noted. Any plans for future pregnancies and views on possible breast feeding should also be obtained. Connective tissue disorders or other autoimmune diseases in either the patient or her family should be recorded.

What is looked for in the physical examination?

The general body habitus is noted and the chest wall examined for any co-existing musculoskeletal deformities. Both breasts are assessed with regard to size, shape, symmetry and the presence or absence of ptosis. The level of each inframammary fold and the distance of each nipple from the sternal notch is recorded. Differences in breast size may necessitate the use of prostheses of different volumes on each side, whilst significant ptosis will not be corrected by augmentation and in some cases may be accentuated. Finally, the nipples are examined and palpation of both breasts performed.

There are neither psychological nor medical contraindications to surgery and the patient wishes to proceed with augmentation. What choices are available concerning the type of prosthesis to be used?

A decision needs to be reached about the size and shape of the prostheses. In addition, as there are differences between prostheses in the nature of the outer shell and the composition of the filling material, a decision must be made on the type of prosthesis to be used. The size is discussed with the patient and this gives the surgeon an opportunity to assess whether or not her expectations of surgery are realistic. Various shapes of prosthesis are available including round and biodimensional prostheses, the latter being designed to produce more fullness in the lower pole of the breast. The most appropriate shape should be chosen by the surgeon depending on the contour of the breast, the shape of the chest wall and the appearance desired by the patient.

The outer shell of prostheses are made of silicone elastomer and may have either a smooth or textured surface. The latter are usually preferred because they are associated with a decreased incidence of capsular contracture.

What are the commonly available filling materials in breast prostheses?

Breast prostheses containing silicone gel were introduced in 1963. This type of prosthesis was used widely until 1992 when the FDA restricted the use of silicone gel to tightly controlled protocols owing to concerns over safety. However, since that date they have continued to be used in many countries including the UK. Saline-inflatable prostheses, where a shell of silicone elastomer is filled with saline peroperatively, remain popular and are currently the most commonly used prostheses in the USA. Trigliceride-filled prostheses contain a filler material derived from soyabean. These were developed more recently to allow better penetration of the augmented breast by X-rays. The manufacturers claim that, if leakage were to occur, the filler material would be absorbed and digested by the body. Anecdotal reports of percutaneous odour from rancid filler material suggest further evaluation of these devices is needed before their use becomes widespread.

Has a link been established between silicone breast prostheses and connective tissue disorders?

A lot of publicity has been given to concerns about the safety of silicone gel breast prostheses. After reviewing all available data, the FDA stated in 1992 that there was no evidence to prove conclusively that there was an association between silicone gel prostheses and any immune disorder. This view was confirmed by a recent UK government sponsored review. However, the media continue to cause anxiety and ignore current scientific evidence.

Silicon (without the final 'e') is a ubiquitous element, the second most abundant element in the earth's crust. In nature, it is bonded to oxygen and occurs in a variety of forms of silica and silicates, and is the main component of sand. Silicone (with the final 'e') is the generic name for a family of synthetic silicon–carbon-based polymers (polydimethyl-siloxane, PDMS) or chains of molecules. Short chains are liquid, progressing to gel, foam and finally a hard resin or rubbery material (elastomer) as the chains increase in length.

The envelopes surrounding breast implants contain very pure *amorphous silica* tightly bonded into the polymer network. Crystalline silica can activate macrophages, stimulate the production of cytokines from macrophages and T-lymphocytes, and enhance the antibody response to foreign protein. However, crystalline silica is not a component of breast implants and its conversion from amorphous silica requires both very high temperatures and catalysts, not conceivable under physiological conditions.

Silicone exposure as a result of bleed from intact implants or even ruptured implants is usually localized to the capsule that forms around the implant. Silicone is hydrophobic, repelling blood and lymph. Silicone has occasionally been identified in lymph nodes after breast or orthopaedic implantation as part of a foreign body reaction. Cadaveric tissue silicone tissue assays have shown elevated levels only within the capsule with levels at different sites, including the spleen and liver, equivalent to baseline levels in non-augmented cadavers.

Exposure to silicone is common and Table 5.1 demonstrates the current medical and non-medical uses of silicone. Since 1990 the media have been terrorising the breast implant population of the world. This has caused considerable anxiety to the extent that some women have even removed their own implants. Implants appear to be guilty until proven innocent. The FDA in America banned the use of implants in 1992 except for use in reconstruction and cosmetic augmentation as part of scientific trials. Saline-filled silicone breast implants and silicone-containing testicular, penile and contraceptive

Table 5.1 Exposure to silicone is common

Non-medical	Medical
Deodorants	Intravenous tubing
Hairsprays	Hypodermic needles
Cosmetics	Syringes
Food	Cerebrospinal fluid shunt tubing
Drinking water	Contraceptive hormone implants
	Testicular prostheses
	Penile implants
	Cardiac valves
	Digital joint arthroplasty prostheses
	Intraocular lens implants

devices are still allowed, as is silicone in food, cosmetics and drugs. Much of the evidence against silicone breast implants published in the literature is anecdotal and of poor epidemiological quality, sometimes with the authors not declaring their conflict of interest. Some have even suggested that the normal scientific process has been hijacked by the legal system. As the results of more rigorous scientifically controlled trials have become available, the balance of favour is swinging back towards the use of silicone implants.

What early post-operative complications may occur?

Haematoma is the most common complication and may require intervention if of significant size. Infection, when it occurs, will generally necessitate removal of the prosthesis. As with any wound there may be delayed healing or a minor degree of wound dehiscence. Numbness of some areas of the breast may be experienced and, in particular, the possibility of altered nipple sensation should be discussed with the patient. This may be either reduced sensation or hypersensitivity. Although in some instances it will be temporary, in some cases it may be permanent.

What late complications should the patient be informed about?

As with any surgery, the scars may be of poor quality. A common complication (up to 40% of cases) is the formation of capsular contracture in relation to the prosthesis. This is in fact a layer of scar tissue which forms around the prosthesis and, if it becomes thick and contracts, it may compress the prosthesis, giving a hard consistency to the breast and altering its shape. There may be associated discomfort for the patient. With the use of textured implants, capsular contracture was reduced in one series at 12 months from 58% with smooth implants to 8% with textured implants. There are few data on the long-term results of capsular excision or capsulotomy following replacement by newer textured implants. Prostheses can also become displaced with time, resulting in a loss of symmetry between the breasts. Wrinkling of the surface of the prosthesis may occur and be visible as rippling under the skin, particularly in the upper part of the breast in very thin patients.

The prosthesis may rupture, resulting in leakage of its contents and loss of volume of the breast. This will usually require another surgical procedure to remove it. The prevalence of rupture of gel-filled prostheses is related to the type of prosthesis used and to the time since the operation. Implants have a finite lifespan, but the average lifespan is not known and will depend on the type. Studies have shown that the first and third generation of implants have very low failure rates but second-generation prostheses have significant leakage rates. Smooth second-generation implants have thin envelopes and have a rupture rate of approximately 10% by 8 years and, by 15 years, the majority of implants of this type are leaking or have ruptured. Newer textured prostheses have an irregular surface, they have a thicker envelope and do not move in the capsule so, unlike smooth prostheses, they are not subjected to shearing forces and friction, and appear much less likely to leak. More recently, a solid silicone gel has been manufactured and is now commonly used as a filler in prostheses, and this gel is considered unlikely to leak. Saline-filled prostheses have a higher risk of deflation and this may occur at any time after surgery.

A complication specific to prostheses filled with silicone gel is that there is often a slow leak of silicone through the outer elastomer shell – a phenomenon known as 'gel bleed'. This has been markedly reduced by changes in the composition of the elastomer shell to produce a more significant barrier. Anyway, the gel bleed is usually intracapsular and only rarely does any silicone leak through the capsule and cause a local inflammatory response with the formation of silicone granulomas. It is almost certainly less likely to occur with the solid silicone gel which is now in widespread use.

Following full discussion of the above, the patient gives informed consent for surgery. What surgical approaches may be used?

The inframammary approach is the most popular, with the incision placed approximately 1 cm above the inframammary crease. The pocket where the prosthesis is to be placed is dissected either directly under the breast and superficial to the pectoral fascia (subglandular plane) or underneath the pectoralis major muscle (submuscular plane). Many surgeons favour submuscular placement in the very thin patient and when using saline prostheses as this provides better soft tissue cover of the prosthesis and lessens the problem of visibility of its margins or any surface rippling. However, a submuscular prosthesis may give a more convex appearance to the upper pole of the breast and there is also on occasion undesirable movements or distortion of the prosthesis when the pectoralis major muscle contracts.

Other approaches include inserting the prosthesis through an axillary, periareolar or even a periumbilical incision. These approaches can be combined with endoscopic instruments to allow small incisions and, providing the patients do not get significant fibrosis in the tunnel between the incision and the breast, they leave minimal visible scarring.

The woman undergoes bilateral augmentation with 200 ml textured silicone gel prostheses which produce an increase in breast measurement to 34B (Figure 5.1b). Post-operative recovery is uneventful. One year later the patient returns complaining of firmness and some discomfort in the right breast. Examination confirms that the right breast has become hard and slightly distorted whilst the left is still soft on palpation. A diagnosis of right-sided capsular contracture is made. What are the treatment options?

Capsular contracture was graded by Baker on a scale of 1–4 according to its severity and only the more severe cases require treatment. Baker has proposed non-surgical treatment with drugs such as papaverine hydrochloride for a trial period of 6 months combined with massage. The practice of closed capsulotomy, which is essentially forceful squeezing of the breast with the aim of rupturing the scar capsule, has now been abandoned owing to the risk of causing rupture of the prosthesis.

Open capsulotomy or capsulectomy may be undertaken and, in such circumstances, the prosthesis is usually replaced. Ultimately, recurrence of severe capsular contracture may require permanent removal of the prosthesis or prostheses.

In the long term is there an increased risk of breast cancer with silicone gel prostheses?

Studies have failed to establish any link between silicone gel prostheses and breast cancer. Two large epidemiological studies at the University of Calgary and the University of California have found no increased incidence of breast cancer in women with silicone prostheses. However, there may be some interference with the detection of early breast cancer by mammography in these patients and special techniques such as the Eklund 'displacement' technique have been suggested for screening.

When undertaking the procedure of breast augmentation, patient selection is the key to success and ensuring a satisfied patient. The patient should have realistic expectations of what can be achieved and an understanding of the potential complications. It is now recommended that all patients receiving breast prostheses have their details entered on to a central register so that outcome data can be regularly reviewed and reported to both patients and the medical profession.

Eight years later, the patient reports a change in shape of the implant. She is concerned about rupture. What techniques are available to assess leakage of silicone and rupture of implants?

Clinical diagnosis of rupture is difficult and imaging is usually required. Several imaging methods including mammography, ultrasonography, computerized tomography (CT) and magnetic resonance imaging (MRI) have been used to assess the integrity of breast implants. Ultrasound is able to image the whole implant and its interior, unlike mammography, and does not involve radiation but is highly operator dependent. The techniques in common use include ultrasound and MRI. Extracapsular spread of silicone gel results in unique sonographic features. A silicone granuloma appears on ultrasonography as a hyperechoic mass with fine internal echoes which extend deep to the posterior wall of the mass and obscures distal structures. This appearance is described on scan as a 'snowstorm' and is highly sensitive for extracapsular rupture. Several other sonographic signs thought to be associated with implant rupture are not as reliable. The collapsed implant shell can sometimes be visualized directly as a series of discontinuous parallel lines described as a 'stepladder' sign, and this is seen in between 32% and 70% of ruptured implants. Central internal echoes within the breast implant were first described as associated with rupture but when present were associated with 55% of rupture in one series and 41% in another. The published estimates of the sensitivity of ultrasonography for implant rupture ranges from 32% to 74%.

In contrast to mammography and ultrasonography, breast MRI accurately depicts both intracapsular and extracapsular rupture. High-resolution MRI is needed to depict the internal structure of implants accurately. When there is extensive leakage of gel, the shell of the implant collapses into the gel and folds in on itself resulting in the 'linguine' sign (Figure 5.2). MRI sensitivity for rupture ranges from 46% to 98%. Studies which have used a dedicated breast coil have reported sensitivities of between 95% and 98%.

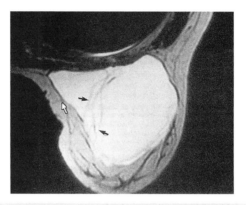

Fig. 5.2 Linguine sign of a ruptured breast implant on a magnetic resonance imaging scan. (The ribbons arrowed represent the wall of the ruptured implant.)

MRI is, however, much more costly than ultrasound. Ultrasound is therefore considered an option as a first investigation for evaluating implant-related complications. What to do with a ruptured implant is not clear. There is widespread agreement that if the implant rupture causes local complications it should be removed with the option of replacement. There is, however, discussion as to whether there is a benefit in removing a ruptured implant that is contained within the scar capsule. Based on the information available in 1992, the FDA recommended that, if an implant is known to be ruptured, it should be removed. At the present time, in the absence of definitive health benefits, widespread screening of breast implant populations is not recommended.

A 16-year-old boy with swelling of his left breast

J R C Sainsbury

A 16-year-old boy presents with a history of swelling of his left breast which has been present for about 6 months. It is very tender and is causing him social embarrassment (Figure 6.1). What is the likely diagnosis and how should it be managed?

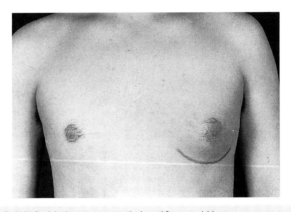

Fig. 6.1 Left-sided gynaecomastia in a 16-year-old boy.

This boy has gynaecomastia. This is benign and usually reverses spontaneously. It is common in puberty and is seen in 30–60% of boys aged 10–16 years. It usually requires no treatment as 80% resolve spontaneously within 2 years. Embarrassment or persistent enlargement are indications for treatment. Symptoms in a boy of this age do not require any specific investigations, although the patient should be carefully examined and the testes checked.

The tenderness is causing significant problems. What treatment options are available?

Studies have suggested that both danazol and tamoxifen are effective in reducing breast swelling and tenderness. Both are effective in about 50% of patients. The dose of danazol is 400 mg a day and the dose of tamoxifen 20 mg a day. There are no randomized studies comparing the two agents. Neither appear to be associated with significant side effects. Body-builders who use anabolic steroids often develop gynaecomastia and a number of these individuals self-prescribe tamoxifen to counteract the oestrogenic effects of the steroids.

Surgery is only indicated when conservative measures fail. The surgical options are liposuction or open surgery to reduce the size of the breast. Liposuction produces few scars but, where there is dense breast tissue, it is not always successful. Ultrasonic liposuction is being developed and appears more effective than simple liposuction. Surgery for gynaecomastia is ideally performed through a circumareolar incision. The aim of the operation should be to leave some breast tissue attached to the back of the nipple and to leave fat on the skin flaps. Otherwise the final cosmetic result can be poor. Only in Klinefelter's syndrome should the aim of surgery be to excise all the breast tissue. Where the breasts are very large, then skin may need to be removed. These latter procedures should be performed by appropriately trained plastic surgeons.

7 A 65-year-old male presents with tender breast swelling

J R C Sainsbury

A 65-year-old man presents with a history of bilateral swelling of both breasts and tenderness on the left side. He is particularly aware of it because his clothes rub against his left nipple which appears very sensitive. What is the likely cause of his symptoms and how should he be managed?

Gynaecomastia is the most likely cause and commonly affects men between the ages of 50 and 80 and, in most cases, does not appear to be associated with any specific endocrine abnormality. There is a need in this age group to exclude other conditions. A careful history and examination may reveal the cause. For instance, the patient may be taking one of a number of drugs or there may be an underlying medical condition. Common causes of gynaecomastia are listed in Table 7.1. A history of recent progressive breast enlargement in the

Table 7.1 Causes of gynaecomastia

Puberty	25%
Idiopathic (senescent)	25%
Drugs (cimetidine, digoxin, spironolactone, androgens or anti-oestrogens)	10–20%
Cirrhosis or malnutrition	8%
Primary hypogonadism	8%
Testicular tumours	3%
Secondary hypogonadism	2%
Hyperthyroidism	1.5%
Renal disease	1%

absence of an easily identifiable cause is an indication for hormonal investigation. If there is concern that the breast enlargement is secondary to obesity, then mammography can differentiate between breast enlargement due to fat or gynaecomastia (Figure 7.1); it is of value if malignancy is suspected. There is no association between gynaecomastia and male breast cancer with the exception of men with Klinefelter's syndrome who are at risk of developing male breast cancer. If there is any clinical or mammographic suspicion of a breast cancer, then fine-needle aspiration cytology or core biopsy should be performed. If there is no clear cause, then blood hormone concentrations should be measured.

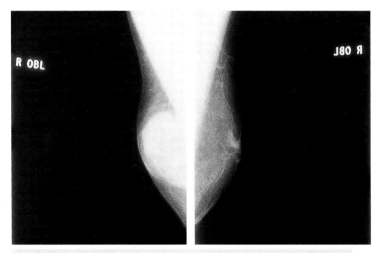

Fig. 7.1 Mammogram showing gynaecomastia.

In idiopathic or senescent gynaecomastia, no specific treatment is required unless symptoms are marked, when tamoxifen or danazol should be considered. Where the cause is drug related, then a change of drug therapy is often effective in reversing the gynaecomastia.

A 29-year-old with severe unilateral breast pain

N J Bundred

A 29-year-old Caucasian woman presents with a 2-month history of severe right-sided breast pain. The pain is associated with tenderness. She stopped the oral contraceptive pill 3 years ago because she developed a deep venous thrombosis. She has two children and has regular menstrual cycles. What features of the pain symptomatology will define the underlying problem? How can you confirm the diagnosis?

The relationship of the pain to her menstrual cycle is important. Cyclical breast pain occurs in 70% of premenopausal women. Breast pain can be separated into two main groups: cyclical and non-cyclical. The best way to assess whether the pain is cyclical is to ask the patient to complete a breast pain record chart (Figure 8.1). Two-thirds of women who report breast pain have cyclical pain and the remaining third have non-cyclical pain. Even in women who have had a hysterectomy if they have had their ovaries conserved it is usually possible to see a pattern of clustering of pain during a certain time each month on the pain chart which indicates a cyclical pattern to the pain. Patients with cyclical pain are by definition premenopausal with an average age of 34. Normal changes which occur in relation to the menstrual cycle include heightened awareness, discomfort, fullness and heaviness of the breasts during the 3–7 days before each period. Women often report areas of tenderness in their breasts and increased breast size at this time. Patients with cyclical breast pain typically suffer increasing severity of pain from mid-cycle onwards with the pain improving at menstruation. The pain is usually described as heavy with the breast being tender to touch and it classically affects the upper outer quadrant of the breast. The pain varies in severity from

Daily Breast Pain Chart

Cyclical Mastalgia

Record the amount of breast pain you experience each day by shading in each box as illustrated

■ Severe pain
◣ Mild pain
• No pain

For example: If you get severe breast pain on the fifth of the month then shade in completely the square under 5. Please note the day your period starts each month with the letter 'P'.

Please bring this card with you on each visit

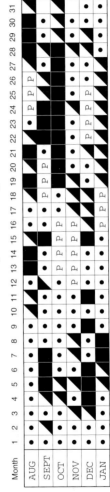

Non-Cyclical Mastalgia

Fig. 8.1 Breast pain chart.

cycle to cycle but can persist for many years. Cyclical mastalgia usually settles at the menopause and post-menopausal women not taking hormone replacement therapy who present with breast pain usually have chest wall pain.

The history suggests the pain is cyclical. What advice would you give this woman?

Thirty per cent of women experience spontaneous resolution of the pain within 6 months of onset. For this reason she should be encouraged to complete a monthly breast pain chart and return for further assessment in 3 months. She should be encouraged to wear a well-supporting bra and she may also gain benefit from wearing the bra at night as well.

The pain does not resolve over the next 3 months and the pain charts demonstrate that the pain is cyclical. How should she be treated?

If the pain has not resolved spontaneously then drug treatment should be instituted (Figure 8.2). Drug treatment should be restricted to patients with pain lasting for more than 7 days per month which persists for more than three cycles. The optimal first-line treatment is gamolenic acid prescribed as evening primrose oil. Each 500 mg capsule of evening primrose oil contains 40 mg of gamolenic acid. It appears that women with severe cyclical mastalgia have low plasma levels of the intermediate metabolites of gamolenic acid which may be due either to inadequate intake or an abnormal metabolism of this compound. In a placebo-controlled trial, gamolenic acid at doses of between 240 and 320 mg per day (between 3–4 g of evening primrose oil per day) improved breast pain, tenderness and nodularity with the maximum benefit occurring after 4 months of treatment. Women should be advised that it does not act as an analgesic and that it can take up to 4 months to determine whether this treatment will be effective. Gamolenic acid in evening primrose oil has a low toxicity and is the optimal initial treatment, especially in younger women wanting to become pregnant or who for those women who may need repeated treatment.

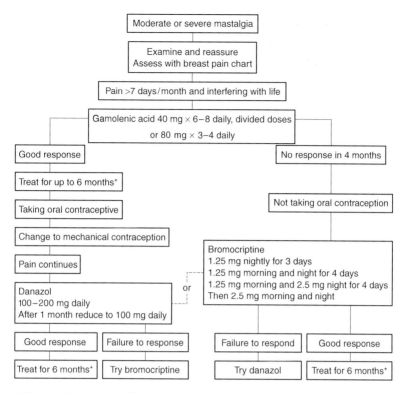

Fig. 8.2 Drug treatment for cyclical mastalgia.

The pain does not resolve after a 4-month course of evening primrose oil. What other options are there for treatment?

Danazol at doses of 100 mg twice a day would normally be the second-choice treatment in a patient with breast pain but it cannot be used in women who have previously had a deep vein thrombosis. If she had been suitable for danazol, then treatment would have been started at a dose of 200 mg per day and given for 1 month. Provided there was a good response, the drug dosage thereafter should be reduced to 100 mg per day. It is often possible to reduce the dose further giving 100 mg daily during days 14–18 of the menstrual cycle or alternatively giving 100 mg every alternate day throughout the menstrual cycle. This limits the unwanted side effects such as menstrual irregularity, weight gain, headache and nausea which affect women taking the higher doses of danazol. Bromocriptine

Table 8.1 Response of cyclical and non-cyclical mastalgia to drug treatment

	Useful response to treatment		
Drug	Cyclical mastalgia	Non-cyclical mastalgia	Side effects
Danazol	79%	40%	30%
Gamolenic acid	58%	38%	4%
Bromocriptine	54%	33%	35%

(2.5 mg daily introduced gradually by increasing the dose over 1–2 weeks) could be prescribed in this patient but it has such a bad side-effect profile (Table 8.1) that many doctors have abandoned its use in this condition. Bromocriptine works because it is a prolactin antagonist. There is a new commercially available prolactin antagonist, cabergoline, which has a very long half-life and so it can be given once a week. It is currently being evaluated for the treatment of breast pain. In view of the fact that this woman cannot take danazol and the problems associated with bromocriptine, the best second-line treatment in this patient is probably tamoxifen in a dose of 10 mg per day. This produces relief of symptoms in approximately 80% of women, although 20% or more suffer severe hot flushes on this treatment. As this drug is not licensed for cyclical breast pain, it should only be prescribed through hospital pain clinics and, even in these clinics, treatment is usually restricted to periods of between 3 and 6 months. It is contraindicated in premenopausal women who are not taking adequate forms of contraception or who are pregnant. Although goserelin, a luteinizing hormone releasing hormone (LHRH) agonist, has been shown in a double-blind crossover trial to be effective in controlling cyclical breast pain, it causes hot flushes and menopausal symptoms. Because it does not have a product licence for this condition, and prolonged use is associated with reduction in bone density, its use should be restricted to specialist breast pain clinics. It is possible to use a combination of goserelin and oestrogen replacement therapy to provide a uniform dose of oestrogen to relieve hot flushes while controlling the breast pain. In the absence of oestrogen, goserelin use should be restricted to a maximum length of treatment of 6 months.

What is the likely response rate?

The response rate to tamoxifen and goserelin is over 80%. The patient should be reviewed 2 months after beginning treatment to assess the response by talking to the patient and checking her pain chart to objectively assess the number of pain-free days. If a clinically useful response has been obtained, treatment can be continued for 6 months but should then be stopped.

After treatment of breast pain with gamolenic acid or the other hormonal agents, pain recurs following a course of treatment in at least half of patients. A repeated course of treatment is not always required because the pain when it does return may not be as severe. A previous failure to respond to a treatment does not preclude a good response to another agent. The response rates to goserelin and tamoxifen remain good, even if a patient has failed to respond to danazol or evening primrose oil. However, if a woman fails to respond to goserelin, she is unlikely to respond to any other agent and consideration should be given as to whether the diagnosis of cyclical pain is correct. Usually further assessment demonstrates the diagnosis was wrong and that the patient has chest wall pain or non-cyclical mastalgia.

9 A 45-year-old woman with pain in the lateral aspect of her breast

N J Bundred

A 45-year-old perimenopausal woman complains of pain in the lateral aspect of her left breast which is constant and not related to her periods. It is severe and she has pain for at least 14 days out of every 28 days of her menstrual cycle. She has recently restarted work as a medical secretary as her children are now at school. She finds the pain disabling and it affects her ability to work. She has already been taking evening primrose oil at a dose of 6 capsules (240 mg) per day for 4 months but this has had no effect on her pain. This woman is concerned that there may be an underlying cause for her pain. What clinical tests would you perform to determine the cause of the pain?

Localized pain in the chest wall, referred pain and diffuse true breast pain must be differentiated (Table 9.1). To determine whether the pain is emanating from the chest wall, the patient should be turned on her

---

Table 9.1 Classification of non-cyclical mastalgia

Chest wall causes
- For example, tender costochondral junctions (Tietze's syndrome)
- Lateral chest wall pain

True breast pain
- Diffuse breast pain
- Trigger spots in breast

Non-breast causes
- Cervical and thoracic spondylosis
- Bornholm disease
- Lung disease
- Gall stones
- Exogenous oestrogens such as hormone replacement therapy
- Thoracic outlet syndrome

---

right-hand side so the breast drops away from the chest wall. In virtually all post-menopausal women presenting with breast pain (except for those on hormone replacement therapy) and in many perimenopausal women, the pain originates from the underlying ribs and muscles with the most common site being in the serratus anterior area. Having rotated the patient into the lateral position, gentle palpation is performed of this area and this often exposes a localized site of chest wall tenderness. If the pain is situated medially, turning the patient on to her side allows the breast to drop away from the costal cartilages and examination at this point allows assessment of whether the pain is originating from the costochondral junction and enables a diagnosis of costochondritis (Tietze's syndrome) to be made.

What is the frequency of non-cyclical breast pain in women presenting with breast pain?

Approximately one-quarter of women presenting with breast pain will have non-cyclical pain and a further 10% have Tietze's syndrome (costochondritis).

Name the two common causes of non-cyclical breast pain.

These are chest wall pain and true non-cyclical breast pain (Table 9.1). It is important to differentiate between these two. The majority of non-cyclical pain is chest wall pain.

How would you manage each type of non-cyclical breast pain?

Improvement of chest wall pain is achieved either by injecting local anaesthetic and steroid (2 ml of 1% lignocaine or marcain combined with 40 mg of methylprednisolone) into the painful area, repeated on two or three occasions if necessary, or by massaging non-steroidal anti-inflammatory gels into the painful area. For a wider area of diffuse chest wall pain, oral non-steroidal anti-inflammatory drugs (e.g. ibuprofen) are given in courses of up to 6 weeks. True non-cyclical breast pain is most frequently subareolar but it also occurs in the medial aspect of the breast and the patient may have some nodularity in this area. Where breast tenderness is associated with non-cyclical breast pain it is important to differentiate between daily pain, which occurs as part of severe continuous cyclical breast pain, from random pain occurring throughout the menstrual cycle with pain-free days in between. Both groups warrant treatment with standard cyclical breast pain drugs such as evening primrose oil, danazol or occasionally tamoxifen. In non-cyclical breast pain the response rate to these agents is lower than that obtained in cyclical breast pain (Table 8.1), but is worth attempting as some patients do get a response. In patients with severe mastalgia who are getting daily pain with no pain-free days, up to 30% get benefits from danazol (Table 8.1). Zoladex and tamoxifen have also been reported to be effective in these patients, although both drugs are unlicensed for this condition and are associated with a greater incidence of side effects than gamolenic acid or danazol. Some women have a localized single tender area in the breast which is known as a trigger spot. Some of these respond to injection of local anaesthetic and steroid. It has been reported that pain can be eliminated in up to half of these women by excision of the trigger spot. However, surgery generally makes breast pain worse and it is well recognized that a number of women develop pain in relation to previous operation scars. Excision of tender painful areas in an attempt to relieve symptoms is therefore rarely appropriate.

A 26-year-old who develops breast tenderness and redness during breast feeding

J M Dixon

A 26-year-old who is 4 weeks post-partum and is currently breast feeding presents with a history that she has had a cracked left nipple of 2 weeks' duration and over the past 24 hours she has developed a localized area of tenderness with some redness of the overlying left breast skin. What is the likely diagnosis and how should you treat it?

This woman is likely to have an infection associated with breast feeding. Lactating infection is often associated with a crack or a break in the skin. This is not the site of entry for organisms into the breast but a break in the skin reduces the body's defence mechanisms against infection and allows increasing numbers of organisms to proliferate on the skin. Lactating infection is usually associated with poor drainage of a segment of the breast, but whether this is the primary event is not clear. The larger than normal number of organisms on the skin enter the duct system and cause infection in the segment of the breast where milk drainage is poor. Treatment of suspected breast lactating infection or puerperal mastitis is oral antibiotics. As the causative organism is usually *Staphylococcus aureus*, the agent of choice is flucloxacillin, 500 mg four times a day, although co-amoxyclav 375 mg three times a day is a reasonable alternative (Table 10.1). If there is a penicillin allergy, erythromycin 500 mg four times a day should be given. Antibiotics that should not be given for breast infection include tetracycline, ciprofloxacin and chloramphenicol as they can all enter the milk and do the child harm. If given early, antibiotics usually control breast infection and stop abscess formation. Each patient should be informed that, if her symptoms do not settle within a week of starting antibiotics, she should return to her primary health care doctor so that she can be referred to hospital for further advice and

Table 10.1 Organisms responsible for and antibiotics most appropriate for treating breast infections

Type of infection	Organism	No allergy to pencillin	Allergy to penicillin
Neonatal	*Staphylococcus aureus* (*Escherichia coli*)*	Flucloxacillin (500 mg four times daily)	Erythromycin (500 mg twice daily)
Lactating	*Staphylococcus aureus* (*Staphylococcus epidermidis*)* (*Streptococci*)*	Flucloxacillin (500 mg four times daily)	Erythromycin (500 mg twice daily)
Non-lactating	*Staphylococcus aureus* Enterococci Anaerobic streptococci *Bacteroides* spp	Co-amoxyclav (375 mg thrice daily)	Combination of erythromycin (500 mg twice daily) with metronidazole (200 mg thrice daily)
Skin associated	*Staphylococcus aureus* (Fungi)*	Flucloxacillin (500 mg four times daily)	Erythromycin (500 mg twice daily)

*Organisms only occasionally responsible.

assessment. Failure of any breast inflammation to settle after a 1-week course of appropriate antibiotics is an indication for urgent hospital referral. While lactating infection occurs most frequently in the first 6 weeks of breast feeding or during weaning it is rarely seen during pregnancy. In contrast, breast cancer can affect women during pregnancy and during the lactating period, and 25% of all breast cancers in women aged less than 35 occur during or within one year of pregnancy (Figure 10.1). There is no evidence that breast cancer occurring during pregnancy or during breast feeding is more aggressive than other breast cancer, but diagnosis is often delayed and

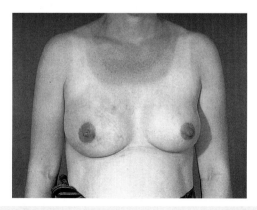

Fig. 10.1 Breast cancer during pregnancy.

so disease is often more advanced at diagnosis with about 65% having involved axillary nodes.

The patient returns a week later and reports that, although initially her symptoms did improve, she has now developed a lump in this area which has become increasingly tender and the skin overlying this area is now erythematous, shiny and thin (Figure 10.2, see colour plate also). What is this patient likely to have developed?

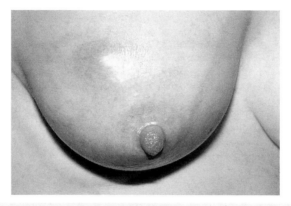

Fig. 10.2 Lactating breast abscess.

She has probably developed a lactating breast abscess. Management of these abscesses has changed over recent years (Figure 10.3). One common form of management is to apply local anaesthetic cream over the affected area and leave this in place for an hour (Figure 10.4). If the skin overlying the abscess is normal, then a needle is inserted into the mass and any pus within the suspected abscess aspirated. Antibiotics are continued and aspiration is repeated every 48–72 hours until no further pus is obtained. If the skin overlying the abscess is thinned,

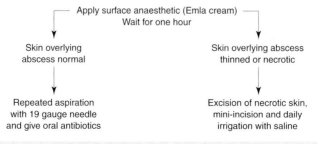

Apply surface anaesthetic (Emla cream)
Wait for one hour

Skin overlying abscess normal

Skin overlying abscess thinned or necrotic

Repeated aspiration with 19 gauge needle and give oral antibiotics

Excision of necrotic skin, mini-incision and daily irrigation with saline

Fig. 10.3 Protocol for treating breast abscesses.

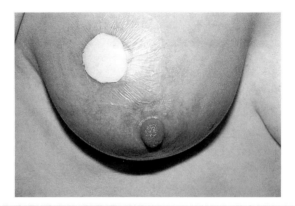

Fig. 10.4 Application of EMLA cream over a lactating abscess.

then a small incision with a 15 blade is made over the point of maximum fluctuance or, if there is necrotic skin, this is excised and the pus is drained. Following incision and drainage, the abscess cavity is irrigated with local anaesthetic, which reduces the pain, and thereafter it is irrigated with normal saline.

Subsequently, irrigation with saline is repeated on a daily basis until the abscess heals. It is not necessary to pack any material into the abscess cavity. Aspiration or mini-incision and drainage (Figures 10.5 and 10.6) results in minimal scarring and both have a high success rate. If having needled a suspected abscess no pus is obtained, a sample of cells should be removed for cytology. Where an abscess is suspected but the diagnosis is not clear, a breast ultrasound scan can be useful to determine whether a localised collection of pus is present.

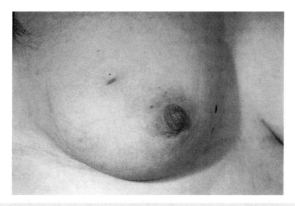

Fig. 10.5 Final cosmetic result following mini-incision and drainage of a lactating abscess.

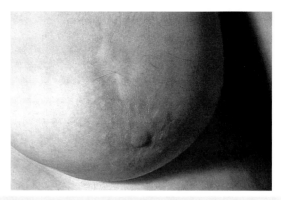

Fig. 10.6 Scars from previous abscess surgery.

Whether the abscess is treated by aspiration, or incision and drainage the patient should be encouraged to breast feed, as this is the best way of draining infected milk from the breast. It has been traditional either to stop patients breast feeding from the affected breast or to use a breast pump. Neither of these approaches are sensible and the baby comes to no harm from drinking infected milk, as the organisms which cause the infection almost certainly originated from the baby's mouth and are killed by gastric acid. Even though flucloxacillin, co-amoxyclav and erythromycin enter breast milk, they will not do the baby any harm. Having had an infection during one pregnancy, patients do not seem more likely to get further infections in subsequent pregnancies.

11 Pain and swelling around the nipple in a 35-year-old

J M Dixon

A 35-year-old woman, who is not lactating, presents with a 1-week history of a painful swelling around her right nipple. She has noticed that the overlying skin is red and inflamed. Treatment with flucloxacillin has produced some improvement in her symptoms, but the pain, erythema and swelling remain. What are the possible diagnoses and what specific questions would you wish to ask this patient?

The most likely diagnosis is periareolar inflammation secondary to periductal mastitis but an inflammatory cancer is also a possible diagnosis. Periductal mastitis occurs almost exclusively in smokers and such patients tend to have recurrent episodes of periareolar infection. In a woman as young as 35 years, if she did have breast cancer, she may have a family history of this disease. The questions which would be relevant to ask are: (1) is she a current smoker or has she previously smoked? (2) has she had any previous similar episodes? and (3) does she have a family history of breast cancer? If so, what was the age of the relative when she developed this? An age of onset less than 40 years in a first-degree maternal relative or a second-degree paternal relative is more likely to indicate a genetic or inherited predisposition and, if this type of family history was present, then breast cancer as a cause of her symptoms would be a real possibility.

Here is a photograph of the patient (Figure 11.1, see colour plate also). What features are present and what would now be your clinical diagnosis?

There is obvious periareolar inflammation without an associated swelling. These features are more in keeping with a diagnosis of

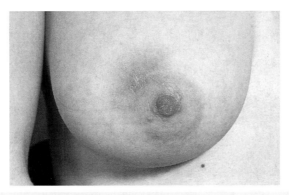

Fig. 11.1 Periareolar inflammation secondary to periductal mastitis.

periductal mastitis than an inflammatory cancer. The lesions of periductal mastitis often contain anaerobic organisms and these patients should be given antibiotics that cover both aerobic and anaerobic bacteria. In a patient who does not have a penicillin allergy, the agent of choice is co-amoxyclav given in a dose of 375 mg three times a day (Table 10.1). If the patient has a penicillin allergy, then a combination of erythromycin and metronidazole should be prescribed. If there is any concern that this lesion is not infective, but an inflammatory cancer, then the lesion should be aspirated and, if solid, a sample of cells sent for cytology.

Following the prescription of co-amoxyclav, the condition resolves, but the patient presents again 3 months later with more florid symptoms and this time there is an obvious tender fluctuant swelling (Figure 11.2, see colour plate also). What has this patient developed and how should she be treated?

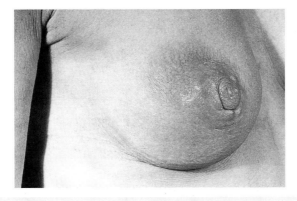

Fig. 11.2 Periareolar abscess secondary to periductal mastitis.

This patient has developed a periareolar abscess. These abscesses occur almost exclusively in patients with periductal mastitis, and are usually due to damage or rupture of a subareolar breast duct. As in the other lesions of periductal mastitis, the organisms responsible for infection can either be aerobic or anaerobic organisms (Table 10.1). Treatment depends on the state of the skin overlying the abscess. If the skin overlying the abscess is normal and not thinned, then following application of local anaesthetic cream (EMLA cream) which is left *in situ* for 1 hour, aspiration to dryness is performed with a white (19 gauge) needle and syringe (Figure 10.4). Pus is sent for bacteriological examination and the patient is given oral co-amoxyclav or erythromycin and metronidazole for 7 days. Patients should be reviewed twice a week and aspiration continued until no further pus is aspirated. If the skin overlying the abscess is thinned, the treatment is as for lactating abscesses with incision and drainage following application of EMLA cream (Figure 10.4). Having drained the pus, the cavity is irrigated, initially with local anaesthetic solution and then normal saline. It is not necessary to pack the abscess cavity and a dry dressing is applied. Thereafter the cavity is irrigated daily with normal saline.

How would the management have differed if the infection had been more peripheral in the breast?

Peripheral non-lactating breast infection is less common than periareolar infection. It is often associated with underlying conditions such as diabetes mellitus, rheumatoid arthritis, steroid treatment, granulomatous lobular mastitis and trauma. Infection associated with granulomatous lobular mastitis can be a particular problem. This condition affects young parous women who may develop large areas of infection with multiple simultaneous peripheral abscesses. These women can present with an inflammatory mass which is indistinguishable from breast cancer. Diagnosis can be made on the basis of fine needle aspiration cytology or core biopsy. There is a strong tendency for this condition to persist and recur and for surgical wounds to drain for a long period of time, and therefore any excision surgery should be avoided in this condition once a diagnosis is established. Although steroids have been tried, there are limited reports of their success. Current management consists of observation and supportive care with surgical intervention being restricted to patients who develop complications such as a breast abscess or a mammary duct fistula.

The organisms responsible for peripheral breast infection are similar to those seen in non-lactating periareolar infection and therefore the antibiotic treatment is the same, and any abscesses are treated by recurrent aspiration or incision and drainage (Table 10.1).

This patient develops recurrent discharge through the site of the drainage wound made to drain the breast abscess (Figure 11.3). What complication has she developed?

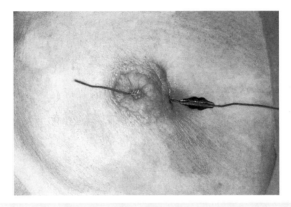

Fig. 11.3 Mammary duct fistula – probe *in situ.*

This patient has developed a mammary duct fistula. Following incision and drainage of a non-lactating periareolar abscess, approximately one-third of patients develop a mammary duct fistula. Such patients have continual discharge of purulent material through the site of abscess drainage. There is a direct communication between the nipple and the skin through a ruptured, damaged breast duct (Figure 11.4) creating a fistula. Treatment of a fistula is excision of the tract incorporating the exit site at the areolar margin and removal of the whole of the involved duct right up to the back of the nipple. As adjacent ducts are often involved by the same process, it is usual to perform a total ductal excision at the same time. Patients should be warned that following excision of the fistula and removal of all ducts from behind the nipple, they may have reduction in nipple sensation. The operation itself is performed under intravenous antibiotic cover, with oral antibiotics being given for 5 days after surgery. It is usually possible to perform

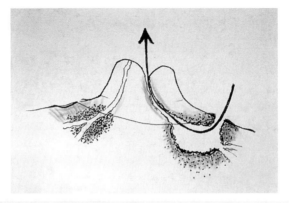

Fig. 11.4 Schematic diagram of a mammary duct fistula.

primary wound closure. Providing the whole of the fistula and diseased duct have been excised, this procedure is associated with a high success rate and when performed through a circumareolar incision produces a satisfactory cosmetic result (Figure 11.5). The previous standard treatment for this condition was to lay open the fistula. Although successful, this produces an ugly scar across the nipple and it is no longer the optimal treatment for this condition.

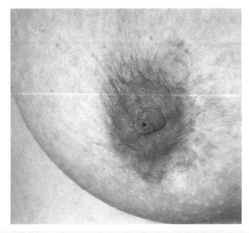

Fig. 11.5 Cosmetic outcome following treatment for a mammary duct fistula.

J M Dixon

A 45-year-old attends with a history of recurrent infection affecting the skin of the lower half of the breast. There is no obvious associated abnormality such as a sebaceous cyst. What are the predisposing factors for this type of infection and what advice would you give her?

Infection affecting the skin of the lower half of the breast is seen most commonly in overweight women with large breasts. The area underneath large breasts becomes hot and sweaty and provides an ideal environment for organisms to proliferate. The increase in the number of organisms permits them to overcome the body's local defence mechanisms and cause infection in the skin. The causative organism is usually *Staphylococcus aureus* (Table 10.1). These infections are more common in women with specific disorders such as diabetes mellitus and hidradenitis suppurativa. Hidradenitis is a condition which affects the apocrine glands of the skin of the axilla, the breast and the groins and is associated with recurrent abscesses and infections at these sites (Figure 12.1).

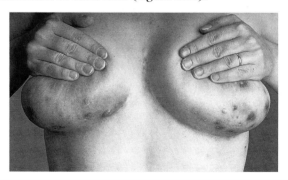

Fig. 12.1 Hidradenitis suppurativa affecting the skin of the lower half of both breasts.

Acute infections should be treated with antibiotics or, if an abscess has developed, with local incision and drainage. Thereafter, providing there is no specific underlying cause, the patient should be given advice about keeping the area as clean and dry as possible. They should be advised to wash this area thoroughly at least twice a day and thereafter to dry the skin carefully either by dabbing with a very soft cotton towel or by using hot air from a hairdryer. No creams or powders should be applied. To keep the area of skin as dry as possible, the patient should wear cotton next to the skin. As some cotton bras are less supportive, an alternative to wearing a cotton bra is to wear a cotton T-shirt or a cotton vest inside the bra. These simple measures are usually effective at reducing the frequency of the infection. In hidradenitis suppurativa, infections should be controlled by a combination of appropriate antibiotics and drainage of any pus (the same organisms are found in hidradenitis as in non-lactating infection – Table 10.1). Conservative excision of the affected skin is effective in stopping further infection in about half of patients, but the remainder have further episodes of infection despite surgery.

Breast lump in a 25-year-old secretary

J R C Sainsbury

**A 25-year-old female medical secretary presents with a 3-month
history of a left breast swelling. She is concerned about the lump
because her great aunt died of breast cancer at the age of 72.
Examination reveals a 2 cm discrete mobile lesion. How would you
investigate this lesion and how would you advise her?**

The most likely diagnosis is a fibroadenoma but, as with all discrete
lesions at any age, a definitive diagnosis needs to be made. All patients
with a breast mass should be assessed by triple assessment (clinical
examination, imaging and fine-needle aspiration cytology). The clinical
examination should take place in a good light with the patient having
her arms by her side, above her head and pressing on her hips. Skin
dimpling or a change in contour is present in a high percentage of
patients with breast cancer (Figure 13.1). Although usually associated
with an underlying malignancy, skin dimpling can follow surgery or

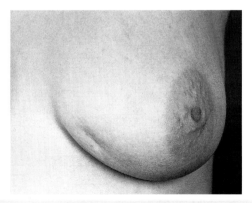

Fig. 13.1 Skin retraction in the lower inner quadrant of the left breast
associated with an underlying breast carcinoma in a 25-year-old.

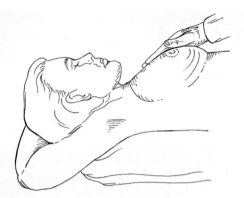

Fig. 13.2 Clinical examination of the breast – position in which breasts should be inspected.

trauma and be associated with benign conditions or it can occur as part of breast involution. The patient has no evidence of dimpling. Breast palpation is performed with the patient lying flat with her arms above or under her head (Figure 13.2). All the breast tissue is examined with the hand held flat. Any abnormality is then further examined with the finger tips and assessed for deep fixation by tensing the pectoralis major, which is accomplished by asking the patient to press on her hips. All palpable lesions should be measured with callipers or by ultrasound, which is more accurate. The lesion in this 25-year-old is discrete, mobile and measures 2 cm in maximum diameter.

Once both breasts have been palpated, nodal areas are checked. Clinical examination of axillary nodes is often inaccurate; palpable nodes can be identified in up to 30% of patients with no clinically significant breast or other disease, and up to 40% of patients with breast cancer who have clinically normal axillary nodes actually have axillary node metastases. The two most commonly used imaging investigations are mammography and ultrasonography. Mammography requires compression of the breast between two breast plates and is often uncomfortable. No nodes are palpable. The standard views are an oblique view and craniocaudal. With modern film screens, a dose of less than 1.5 mGy is standard. Mammography allows detection of mass lesions, areas of parenchymal distortion and microcalcification. Because breasts are relatively radiodense in women aged under 35, mammography is rarely of value in this age group.

In ultrasonography, high-frequency sound waves are beamed through the breast and the reflections detected and turned into images. Cysts show up as transparent objects and other benign lesions tend to have well-demarcated edges whereas cancers usually have indistinct outlines. An ultrasound shows a $16 \times 12 \times 8$ mm well-defined solid benign lesion.

Fine-needle aspiration can differentiate between solid and cystic lesions. Aspiration of solid lesions requires skill to obtain sufficient cells for cytological analysis and expertise is needed to interpret these smears. In some centres, cytopathologists take the specimen, but aspiration is usually performed by a clinician. A 21 or 23 gauge needle is attached to a syringe which is used with or without a syringe holder. The needle is introduced into the lesion and suction is applied by withdrawing the plunger; multiple passes are made through the lesion before the plunger is released and the needle withdrawn. The material in the needle and syringe is then spread on to microscope slides. The slides are either dried or sprayed with an alcohol fixative, depending on the cytologist's preference and are stained. It is possible for the smears to be reported immediately. Cytology of the lump is reported as showing features of a fibroadenoma.

False-positive results occur as with any diagnostic techniques. The accuracy of investigations used in the diagnosis of breast lumps is outlined in Table 13.1. It is routine to plan treatment on the basis of malignant cytology supported by a diagnosis of malignancy on clinical examination and imaging. Cytology has a false-positive rate of about 2 per 1000, and the lesions most likely to be misinterpreted are fibroadenomas and areas of the breast which have been irradiated. The

Table 13.1 Accuracy of investigations in diagnosis of symptomatic breast disease in specialist breast clinics

	Clinical examination	Mammography	Ultrasonography	Fine-needle aspiration cytology
Sensitivity for cancers*	86%	86%	82%	95%
Specificity for benign disease†	90%	90%	85%	95%
Positive predictive value for cancers§	95%	95%	90%	99.8%

*Of cancers detected by test as malignant or probably malignant (that is, complete sensitivity).
†Of benign disease detected by test as benign.
§Of lesions diagnosed as malignant by test that are cancers (that is, absolute positive predictive value).

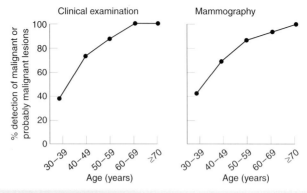

Fig. 13.3 Sensitivity of clinical examination and mammography by age in patients presenting with a breast mass. (From: Dixon JM. ABC of Breast Diseases. London: BMJ Publishing Group 1995; p. 4, with permission.)

sensitivity of clinical examination and mammography varies with age and only two-thirds of cancer in women aged under 50 are considered suspicious or definitely malignant on clinical examination or mammography (Figure 13.3).

In women aged under the age of 35, triple assessment consists of clinical examination, ultrasonography and fine-needle aspiration cytology, with the substitution or addition of mammography in women over the age of 35. In one series of 1511 patients with breast cancer having triple assessment, only six patients (0.2%) had lesions considered to be benign on all three investigations.

The role of cytology in the investigation of a breast mass is outlined in Figure 13.4. An alternative to cytology is to remove a small core of tissue from the mass by means of a cutting needle technique. A 14 gauge needle is used with an automatic biopsy gun to allow the procedure to be performed single handed. This breast mass has a sensitivity of approximately 95%.

In a female aged 25, a fibroadenoma is the most common cause of a discrete lump and all investigations were consistent with this diagnosis (Figure 13.5). Fibroadenomas account for 60% of discrete lumps in women aged 20 or younger and comprise about 13% of all symptomatic breast masses. They present as discrete breast masses which can be single or multiple, and decrease in frequency with age. On ultrasound, fibroadenomas have well-defined margins with a heterogeneous echo pattern. Ultrasound allows assessment of size (Figure 13.6). Cytological examination can confirm the diagnosis and a

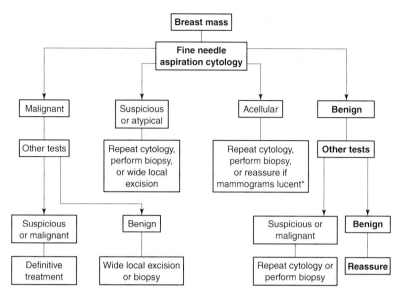

* An acellular cytological report is acceptable in the presence of lucent mammograms.

Fig. 13.4 Investigation of a breast mass.

fibroadenoma is characterized cytologically by sheets of benign
epithelial cells in a background of bare nuclei. A core biopsy may be
indicated if atypical cells are reported on cytology or in patients with a
strong family history where a definitive histological diagnosis is
required. The only real differential diagnosis in a female of this age is
an area of benign breast change. If the patient had been 40 years of age
with the same mass then the differential diagnosis would have
included a phyllodes tumour and malignancy.

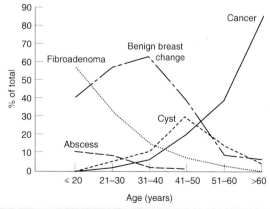

Fig. 13.5 Changing frequencies of different discrete breast lumps with age.
(From: Dixon JM. ABC of Breast Diseases. London: BMJ Publishing Group
1995; p. 8, with permission.)

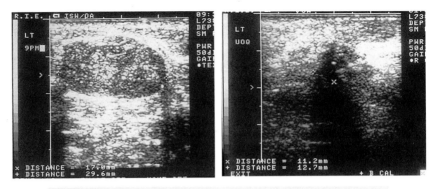

Fig. 13.6 Fibroadenoma on ultrasound. Compare the differences with cancer, seen on the right.

Simple fibroadenomas are not associated with any significant malignant potential, although complex fibroadenomas (those associated with surrounding proliferative changes) are associated with a slight but not significant increased risk of breast cancer. Although classified in most textbooks as benign neoplasms, fibroadenomas are best considered as aberrations of normal development (Table 13.2) as they develop from a whole lobule and not from a single cell. They are very common and are under the same hormonal control as the remainder of the breast tissue. There are four different type of fibroadenomas: the common fibroadenoma, giant fibroadenoma, juvenile fibroadenoma and phyllodes tumours. There is no universally accepted definition of what constitutes a giant fibroadenoma, but most consider that a giant fibroadenoma should measure over 5 cm. Juvenile fibroadenomas (Figure 13.7) occur in adolescent girls and sometimes undergo rapid growth, but are managed in exactly the same way as the

Table 13.2 Aberrations of normal development and involution

Age (years)	Normal process	Aberration
<25	Breast development	
	Lobular	Fibroadenoma
	Stromal	Juvenile hypertrophy
25–40	Cyclical activity	Cyclical mastalgia
		Cyclical nodularity (diffuse or focal)
35–55	Involution	
	Lobular	Macrocysts
	Stromal	Sclerosing lesions
	Ductal	Duct ectasia

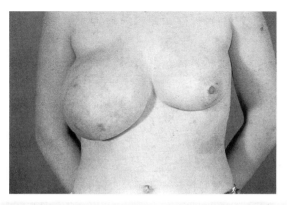

Fig. 13.7 Juvenile fibroadenoma.

common fibroadenoma. Phyllodes tumours are distinct pathological entities and cannot always be differentiated clinically from fibroadenomas.

Current evidence of the natural course of fibroadenomas suggests that less than 10% of them increase in size and about one-third become smaller or disappear. Fibroadenomas, therefore, do not of necessity need excision and an observational policy may suffice. Repeat measurements are possible with ultrasound. Excision or obtaining a histological diagnosis by core biopsy is indicated if the lesion is growing on ultrasound, if it is 3 cm or greater in size, if there is any suspicion or atypia on cytology, or if the patient requests this. Excision, once a definitive diagnosis has been established, can usually be performed either through a circumareolar incision or an axillary skin crease incision with tunnelling between the subcutaneous and breast fat to directly over the lesion. Care must be taken not to damage the subcutaneous fat along the tunnel as this can result in post-operative skin dimpling. Excision in the plane of the capsule of a fibroadenoma avoiding removal of any normal surrounding breast tissue will allow even the largest fibroadenoma to be removed without creating a defect in the breast.

The family history is irrelevant in this case as her great aunt is too distant a relative and she was elderly when she developed breast cancer. If the family history had been much stronger, and she had one or more first degree relatives who developed breast cancer under the age of 40, then the most sensible approach would be to advise excision. An alternative would be to obtain a definitive diagnosis by performing a core biopsy.

A 23-year-old presents with recent onset breast asymmetry

J M Dixon

A 23-year-old woman presents with a short history that she has noticed marked breast asymmetry and she feels there is a large mobile lump in her left breast. The clinical photograph taken at the time she was seen is shown (Figure 14.1). What are the clinical features present and what is the likely diagnosis?

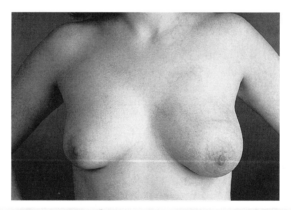

Fig. 14.1 Giant fibroadenoma.

There is marked breast asymmetry with the left breast obviously being larger than the right. There are very prominent veins over the skin of the left breast and the skin looks stretched. The likely diagnosis is of a juvenile or giant fibroadenoma.

How would you confirm this diagnosis?

Clinically a giant or juvenile fibroadenoma is well circumscribed and mobile. It must be differentiated from a phyllodes tumour which tends to affect older women, the mean age of women with this condition being between 40 and 50 years. Phyllodes tumours are seen in younger women but are uncommon. Juvenile fibroadenomas are characteristically seen in teenagers or in women in their early 20s. The investigation of choice in such a large lesion is a core biopsy and this should be performed to confirm the diagnosis.

The core biopsy suggests the lesion is a juvenile fibroadenoma. How would you approach the lesion to remove it?

The classical approach is a submammary incision just above the inframammary fold. Having deepened the incision, the breast is then elevated off the chest wall and the lesion is removed from behind. An alternative is an approach through an inferolateral incision, similar to the incision used for breast augmentation. It is not usually necessary to make the incision as large as the lesion. In histologically proven juvenile or giant fibroadenomas the lesions are shelled out from surrounding tissue and, providing the lesion is removed entirely, recurrence is not a problem. Delivery of a large fibroadenoma through a wound which is smaller than the size of the lesion can be awkward but is usually possible. The incision is deepened and then developed out laterally to the edge of the breast. The breast is reflected off the pectoral fascia and the fibroadenoma is removed through the deep surface of the breast.

This particular fibroadenoma measured over 9 cm (Figure 14.2). There is often concern, because of the extra skin present over the lesion, that

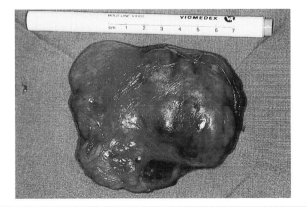

Fig. 14.2 Operative specimen of a giant fibroadenoma (from Figure 14.1).

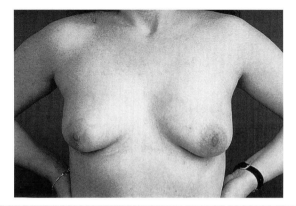

Fig. 14.3 Cosmetic result after excision of a giant fibroadenoma.

once the breast mass is removed this excess skin will remain. As in the patient illustrated, the breast usually returns to a normal shape and the excess skin retracts (Figure 14.3). Furthermore, because of the use of an inferolateral approach, no scar is visible. The plan in such women should be to remove the juvenile or giant fibroadenoma and wait a few months to assess whether the skin, breast contour and volume return to normal. If the cosmetic result is unsatisfactory after 3 months, then the patient should be referred for a plastic surgical opinion and be considered for a mastopexy.

A 45-year-old woman with a history of a phyllodes tumour presents with a further breast lump

J R C Sainsbury

A 45-year-old woman reports that 4 years ago she had a 8 cm benign phyllodes tumour excised from her left breast. She has become aware of a further lesion deep to the scar. What is the likely cause of her lump and how would you establish a diagnosis?

It is probable that she has a recurrence of her phyllodes tumour. If the original phyllodes tumour was visible on mammograms, then mammography might confirm the presence of a recurrent lesion (Figure 15.1). It would be important to have the original pathology reviewed to ensure that the lesion had been completed excised at the first operation and that it was considered to be at the benign end of

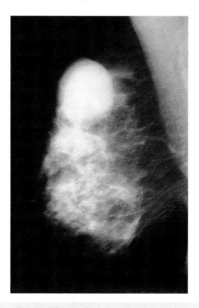

Fig. 15.1 Mammogram of a phyllodes tumour.

the spectrum of these lesions. A recurrent phyllodes tumour can be confirmed by core biopsy.

How should this patient be treated?

The patient needs a further excision. As there has been one recurrence, it is important that the recurrent lesion is excised with a good margin of surrounding breast tissue. This means that approximately 1–2 cm of normal breast tissue should be removed. Recurrent phyllodes tumours may be best treated by subcutaneous mastectomy and immediate reconstruction.

A 19-year-old with a history of treatment for malignant phyllodes tumour who presents with a rapidly enlarging breast

J R C Sainsbury and J M Dixon

A 19-year-old is referred from another hospital. She was initially seen 3 months prior to referral with a 10 cm discrete mobile mass in the left breast. No pre-operative investigations were performed and a presumptive diagnosis of a juvenile fibroadenoma was made in view of her age. The lesion was shelled out through a circumareolar incision with a lateral extension. Subsequent pathology suggested a malignant phyllodes tumour. This is unusual in such a young patient. She now presents with a rapidly enlarging left breast (Figure 16.1, see colour plate also). What are the features that are present? How do benign and malignant phyllodes tumour differ histologically?

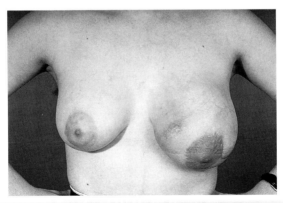

Fig. 16.1 Patient with a recurrent malignant phyllodes tumour in the left breast.

The features that are present are that the left breast is grossly distended and much larger than the right. There are very prominent veins over the breast and there is visible tumour supramedially which is stretching the overlying skin.

Phyllodes tumours have two elements: stroma and epithelium. The features used to differentiate between benign and malignant phyllodes tumours include cellular atypia, mitotic activity and tumour margin. Using combined criteria, a phyllodes tumour is classified as benign if there are 0–4 mitoses in 10 high-powered fields, borderline if there are 5–9 mitoses in 10 high-powered fields or infiltrating margins and minimal stromal cellular atypia, or malignant if there are 10 or more mitoses in 10 high-powered fields, infiltrating margins or moderate to marked stromal cellular atypia. Metastases occur only in association with malignant tumours but, even with this classification, only approximately one-quarter of patients diagnosed as having a malignant phyllodes tumour will develop metastatic disease. The origin of phyllodes tumours is not clear but the lesion probably arises *de novo* from breast parenchyma rather than arising from a pre-existing fibroadenoma.

Are there any other investigations you would perform in this patient before considering surgery?

Malignant phyllodes tumours rarely metastasize but, when they do, the most common site for metastasis is lung. In such a large tumour (there were two palpable masses in this patient, one 12×10 cm and the other 8×8 cm) it is appropriate to screen for lung metastases by performing a chest X-ray and CT scan of the thorax.

The CT scan is clear. How would you treat her?

This girl requires a mastectomy and, in view of her age, it would be appropriate to perform immediate reconstruction. It is important during the dissection that the tumour is removed intact. To do this, it will be necessary to remove skin over the tumour medially. Mastectomy would need to incorporate the area of abnormal skin. Phyllodes tumours do not normally metastasize to lymph nodes as they are sarcomas rather than carcinomas. Reconstruction could be either with a latissimus dorsi (LD) or transverse rectus abdominis myocutaneous (TRAM) flap. If a latissimus dorsi flap is used, then an implant would be needed. For some large tumours a flap is necessary for skin cover and immediate reconstruction is not possible (Figures 16.2a and b).

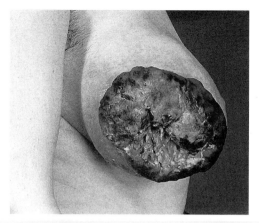

Fig. 16.2(a) Malignant phyllodes tumour.

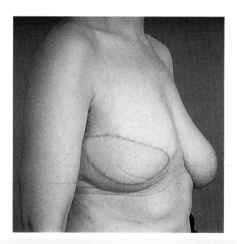

Fig. 16.2(b) Following excision and LD flap.

What is the role of adjuvant therapy in malignant phyllodes tumours?

There are no clear data from the literature on the role of adjuvant radiotherapy or chemotherapy in this situation. In such a large lesion, chest wall radiotherapy is often given empirically. There is no role at the present time for routine adjuvant chemotherapy in this situation. If metastases are present, then an anthracycline-containing regime would be most appropriate.

J R C Sainsbury

Mrs C is 47 years old and presents with a 4-day history of having developed a large breast lump which she discovered in the shower. She has regular menstrual cycles and there is no family history of breast cancer. She is adamant that the lump has not been present for longer than a few days. Her husband reports that he can see the lump. What is the likely diagnosis. How would you confirm this and what further information would you elicit?

Any discrete lump presenting suddenly in a woman in her late 40s is likely to be a cyst (Figure 17.1). Cysts are anechoic on ultrasound and have a characteristic halo on mammography. Most present as a smooth discrete breast lump that can be painful and sometimes can be visible. For symptomatic cysts the diagnosis is confirmed by needle aspiration.

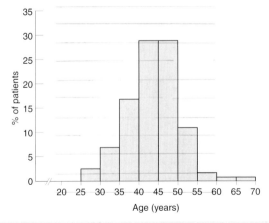

Fig. 17.1 Age distribution of cysts. (Adapted from Haagensen CD, Bodian C, Haagensen DE. Breast Carcinoma Risk and Detection. Philadelphia: WB Saunders, 1981.)

Cysts often precede the menstrual irregularity associated with the menopause by 5 years and ascertaining the age of the mother's menopause often confirms this. They are most common in the 40–50 year age group (Figure 17.1). They represent part of the process of involution (Table 13.2). Breast involution begins sometime after the age of 30. During involution the breast stroma is replaced by fat so that the breast becomes less radiodense, softer and ptotic. Changes in the glandular tissue include the development of areas of fibrosis, the formation of small cysts (microcysts) and an increase in the number of glandular elements (adenosis). Palpable breast cysts are aberrations of the involutional process (Table 13.2). Mammography should be performed if it has not previously been carried out within the last 12 months as between 1 and 3% of patients with cysts have carcinomas; few of these cancers are directly associated with the cyst (Figure 17.2). Aspirated cyst fluid is discarded if clear or uniformly coloured and only if it is bloodstained should it be sent for cytology. If a lump persists post-aspiration, then the lump should be investigated by ultrasound and, if solid, fine-needle aspiration cytology. The use of ultrasound at the time of aspiration allows confirmation of complete aspiration and enables assessment of any other lesions visible on mammography. Indications for excision of a cyst are obtaining bloodstained fluid after a non-traumatic aspiration, a residual mass following aspiration of fluid and persistent refilling of the same cyst over a short time interval.

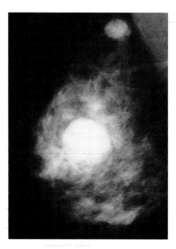

Fig. 17.2 Mammogram of an intracystic cancer. Note the irregular hypoechoic lesion (cyst) centrally with the irregular solid lesion lining the mass.

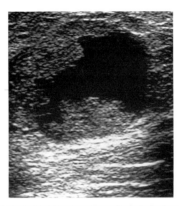

Fig. 17.3 Ultrasound of an intracystic carcinoma.

Needle biopsy techniques are of limited use in these situations as they do not reliably distinguish between intracystic papillomas and low-grade intracystic papillary carcinomas. Ultrasound can visualize such lesions (Figure 17.3) and allow image-guided core biopsy to confirm the diagnosis.

How common are cysts?

Approximately 7% of women in the Western world present at some time during their lifetime with a palpable breast cyst. Cysts were first distinguished as separate entities in 1829 by Astley Cooper. Approximately half of all women who present with a palpable breast cyst will only ever have one symptomatic palpable cyst, a third will develop between two and five, and one in six will develop more than five cysts. Two per cent of women will have more than 25 palpable cysts and 1% will have more than 100. Cysts usually disappear at the menopause and, until recently, palpable cysts developing in women over the age of 50 were uncommon. With the use of hormone replacement therapy (HRT), it is now no longer uncommon to see cysts in older women. Women who develop palpable breast cysts prior to the menopause will usually continue to have cysts on HRT. Cysts which have disappeared prior to starting HRT will often reappear. Not all cysts need to be aspirated and, in patients with multiple cysts, it is inappropriate to aspirate the many cysts that are present in these women's breasts. As ultrasound is as sensitive and specific for a diagnosis of a cyst as aspiration, palpable breast masses should be marked and, once confirmed as cysts, should only be aspirated if symptomatic. Danazol has been reported to reduce cyst formation and can be used in patients with multiple cysts.

Is there an association between cysts and breast cancer?

The published evidence relating breast cysts and breast cancer is confusing and conflicting. The major reason is that different authors have used different definitions of cystic disease. Those studies that have included only patients presenting with clinically palpable cysts have consistently shown that these women are much more likely than the general population to develop breast cancer (Table 17.1). The increased risk in these women in the studies summarized in Table 17.1 ranges from 1.7 to 7.5 times that of the normal population. The largest and most recent study reported included 1374 women with palpable cysts and indicated that women with cysts were 3.25 times more likely to develop breast cancer than women without cysts. This risk appeared to be highest in women who develop cysts under the age of 45. It also showed that the increased risk persisted and was still present more than 5 years after cyst aspiration. As there are no proven screening techniques in these younger women at the present time, it is not recommended that they are screened more frequently or at a younger age than that currently provided by recognized screening programmes.

Table 17.1 Incidence of breast cancer in women with palpable breast cysts

Author	Year	Number of women	Follow-up (years)	Number of cancers	Relative risk
Chardot	1970	206	5	6	7.5
Haagensen	1984	2511	5–30	72	2.48
Roberts et al.	1984	428	10–15	17	3.5
Jones and Bradbeer	1980	332	5	7	2.5
Harrington and Lesnick	1980	596	5.6	19	3.5
Ciatto et al.	1990	3809	1–7	34	1.77
Bundred et al.	1991	352	5–12	14	4.4
Bruzzi et al.	1997	802	6	17	1.69
Dixon et al.	1998	1374	9.4	65	3.24

The first three studies listed included patients with cystic disease diagnosed by biopsy and aspiration, whereas the remaining studies include only patients diagnosed by aspiration.

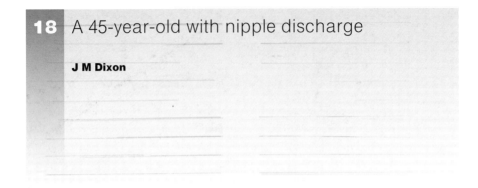

18 A 45-year-old with nipple discharge

J M Dixon

A 45-year-old reports that she has noticed a very localized discharge from her nipple. What specific questions would you ask her?

It is important to know the colour of the discharge, the frequency of the discharge, and whether it is spontaneous or is present only on squeezing the nipple. Discharge associated with serious underlying pathology is usually spontaneous, bloodstained or persistent. Approximately two-thirds of non-pregnant women will produce nipple discharge if the nipple is cleaned and suction applied to the nipple. This normal or physiological discharge varies in colour from white to pale yellow to green to a blue black colour. Characteristically it comes from multiple ducts and is rarely spontaneous. The majority of patients sent up to hospital with what is described as galactorrhoea actually have white-coloured physiological discharge. Patients with galactorrhoea spontaneously produce large amounts of fluid and, when squeezed, milk jets out of the nipple.

What features should you look for on examination?

Some patients who present with nipple discharge do not have discharge from the breast ducts but have discharge from the surface of the nipple or the areola. These areas should therefore be carefully examined as discharge from the nipple is one mode of presentation of Paget's disease or nipple eczema. Paget's disease can usually be differentiated from nipple eczema because Paget's disease always affects the nipple (Figure 18.1, see colour plate also), there is loss of surface epithelium centrally and it only affects the areola thereafter. In contrast, eczema principally affects the areola and spreads on to the

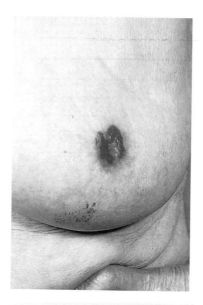

Fig. 18.1 Paget's disease of the nipple.

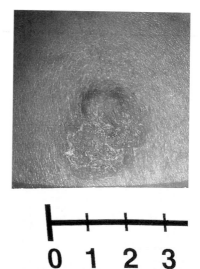

Fig. 18.2 Eczema of the nipple.

nipple only as a secondary event (Figure 18.2, see colour plate also). If there is a lesion affecting the nipple and areola but there is doubt about the diagnosis, then either scrapings of the abnormal skin should be sent for cytology or a portion of the abnormal skin should be removed under local anaesthetic and sent for histologic assessment.

Having established that the nipple/areola complex looks normal, a clinical examination should be performed to determine if there is an associated mass. Attempts should then be made to produce the discharge by squeezing the nipple. A careful note should be taken of whether the discharge emanates from a single or multiple ducts, and whether it is unilateral or bilateral; details of colour and whether the discharge is obviously bloodstained should also be recorded. If a discharge is obtained by squeezing the nipple, but it is not obviously bloodstained, it should be tested for the presence or absence of blood using a commercial Stix preparation. While this is useful, these areas are very sensitive and anything other than gentle squeezing of the nipple to produce the discharge will produce a positive test for blood.

How is nipple discharge investigated and managed?

Patients should have a full clinical examination and, if over the age of 35, they should have a mammogram. If there is either a mass present

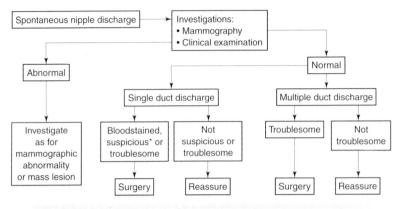

Fig. 18.3 Investigation of nipple discharge.

or if a suspicious mammographic abnormality is identified, then this should be appropriately investigated (Figure 18.3). Otherwise, patients who have no clinical abnormality on clinical or mammographic examination are managed according to whether their discharge is from a single or multiple ducts. Indications for surgery are a single duct discharge which is bloodstained, persistent or troublesome; multiple duct discharge normally requires surgery only when it is causing the patient trouble (Figure 18.3). Patients with true galactorrhoea should have a careful drug history taken as a number of drugs, particularly psychotropic drugs, cause hyperprolactinaemia. Blood should be taken for prolactin and, where prolactin levels are elevated, then a search for a pituitary tumour should be instituted.

When planning the site of incision for removal of a single duct (microdochectomy), it is useful to identify the direction of the diseased duct by pressing around the nipple over the areola, as pressure over the dilated duct produces discharge from the nipple. A probe is placed in the discharging duct at the start of the operation to assist identification of the abnormal duct. A circumareolar incision is then made either over the site where pressure produces discharge or directly over where the probe is palpated and, having deepened the incision, dissection is continued under the areola until the dilated duct containing the probe is identified. As most lesions which cause duct discharge affect the distal 2 cm of the duct, this is the total length of duct which needs to be excised in the majority of patients. Galactography or ductography are of limited utility in the evaluation of nipple discharge. A normal galactogram does not reliably exclude the presence of intraductal pathology in a patient with symptoms, suggesting an underlying pathologic cause. However, in a young woman who wants to preserve the ability to breast feed, a pre-operative galactogram which localizes the filling defect can allow excision of a minimal amount of the ductal system.

The most common cause of a bloodstained nipple discharge is a duct papilloma and less than 5% of bloodstained nipple discharges are actually related to breast cancer (Figure 18.4, see colour plate also).

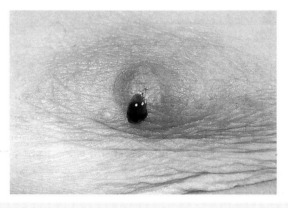

Fig. 18.4 Bloodstained nipple discharge.

If the discharge is from multiple ducts and is thick or cheesy, what is the likely diagnosis?

The major subareolar ducts dilate and shorten during involution and, by the age of 70, 40% of women have substantial duct dilatation. Clinically this is known as duct ectasia and it is probably no more than simple involution of the breast ducts, but some women have excessive dilatation and shortening of the ducts, and develop nipple discharge or nipple retraction. This is an aberration of the normal involutional process (Table 13.2). The discharge is usually cheesy and the nipple retraction is usually slit-like (Figure 18.5). Surgery is indicated if the discharge is troublesome or if the patient wishes the nipple to be everted. Surgery involves removing all the ducts underneath the nipple (a total duct excision). This is performed through a small circumareolar incision based at 6 o'clock. Patients should be warned that following this operation there can be changes in nipple sensitivity:

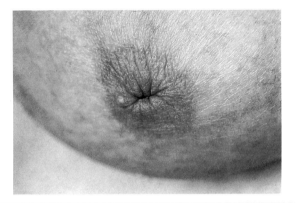

Fig. 18.5 Slit-like nipple retraction due to duct ectasia.

the nipple may become less sensitive in up to a third of women and more sensitive in approximately one-quarter.

You suspect Paget's disease. How would you manage this patient?

All patients with suspected Paget's disease should have a careful clinical examination and mammography. If a nipple biopsy confirms Paget's disease and there is no clinical or mammographic mass, the standard treatment until recently has been mastectomy. The majority of these patients will be found on pathology to have ductal carcinoma *in situ* affecting the subareolar ducts with or without an associated invasive focus. Some patients have microcalcification visible on mammography underneath the nipple at the site of the carcinoma *in situ*. It is possible to confirm that this microcalcification is associated with carcinoma *in situ* by performing an image-guided core biopsy. In patients with either no clinical mass or mammographic evidence suggestive of carcinoma *in situ* in continuity with the nipple, a wide excision of the nipple/areola complex and the underlying ducts followed by post-operative radiotherapy produces satisfactory long-term local control rates providing that the excision margins are free of disease. This has now replaced mastectomy in many centres as the treatment of choice for this condition. Patients with Paget's disease and a palpable mass lesion which is shown on investigation to be an invasive breast cancer usually require a mastectomy unless the lesion is situated directly underneath the nipple when a wide excision of the mass and nipple/areolar complex and post-operative radiotherapy is an option. Paget's disease is associated with 1–2% of all breast cancers.

If the clinical or histological diagnosis is eczema, then this is treated with local steroid application; 1% hydrocortisone applied twice a day is usually effective. Patients should also be given advice about washing their bras separately in hypoallergenic washing powder or they should be advised to wear a pad between the bra and nipple/areola skin to avoid potential allergens affecting this area.

Recent onset nipple inversion/retraction in a 55-year-old woman

J M Dixon

A 55-year-old presents with a history that she has noticed her nipple has become pulled in. How would you investigate her and what are the possible causes?

Causes of nipple retraction include benign disease such as duct ectasia, periductal mastitis and tuberculosis. It could also be iatrogenic and follow previous surgery. Slit-like retraction of the nipple as shown on Figure 18.5 is characteristic of benign disease. If the whole nipple is pulled in (Figure 19.1), then causes include breast cancer or inflammatory breast conditions such as periductal mastitis. Nipple retraction can also be congenital. Investigation of a patient with acquired nipple retraction is outlined below (Figure 19.2).

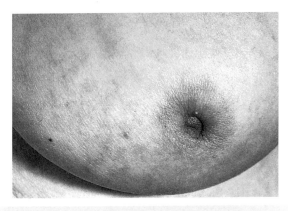

Fig. 19.1 Nipple retraction due to breast cancer.

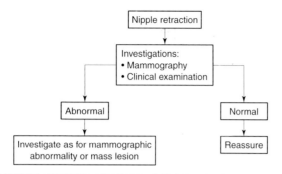

Fig. 19.2 Investigation of nipple retraction.

Some women find congenital or acquired nipple retraction distressing. What can be done to treat this symptom?

Nipple shields and suction devices are available to try and evert nipples but they rarely produce long-term benefit. Failure of these devices is due to the major ducts being shortened either as a developmental anomaly or as a result of disease, most commonly periductal mastitis. It is possible surgically to evert these nipples but this requires division of the breast ducts (Figures 19.3a and b). Although this produces satisfactory cosmetic results, it does mean that the patient cannot breast feed and there is the slight risk that, following such operations, nipple sensation is reduced.

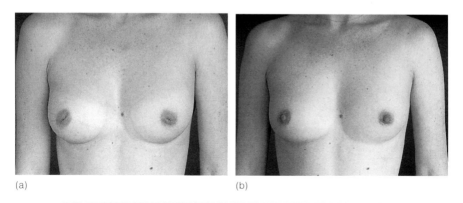

(a)   (b)

Fig. 19.3 Photograph of a patient with nipple retraction (a) before and (b) after surgery to evert the nipple.

20 A woman at increased risk of breast cancer due to family history

M Morrow

A 35-year-old woman is referred by her general practitioner for a breast cancer risk evaluation. Her mother had unilateral breast cancer at age 40. One maternal aunt had bilateral breast cancer, the first cancer developing at age 45 and the second at age 62, and a second maternal aunt had unilateral breast carcinoma at age 66. Two other maternal aunts, age 65 and 70 have never had breast cancer, and the patient has one unaffected sister age 28. Her maternal grandmother died at age 40 in an automobile accident. There is no family history of ovarian cancer. Is this patient an appropriate candidate for genetic screening?

Mutation in a breast cancer predisposition gene is an uncommon cause of breast cancer thought to account for approximately 10% of cases. Genetic breast cancer is suspected when three or more relatives on the same side of the family tree have had breast cancer, or when the combination of breast and ovarian cancer is seen. Breast cancer with an early age of onset, bilateral breast cancer and a pattern consistent with autosomal dominant inheritance increase the level of suspicion that a genetic mutation may be present. Breast cancer susceptibility is generally inherited as an autosomal dominant with limited penetrance. This means that it can be transmitted through either sex and some family members may transmit the abnormal gene without developing breast cancer themselves. It is not yet known how many breast cancer genes there are. This 35-year-old woman has four affected relatives, two who had early-onset breast cancer and one who has had bilateral disease, and so she is clearly at risk of developing breast cancer. To understand the options for genetic testing, one needs a detailed knowledge of the genetics of breast cancer.

Just over a third of familial cases of breast cancer are thought to occur due to a mutation in the first breast cancer gene discovered, BRCA1, which is on the long arm of chromosome 17. BRCA1 is a large gene spanning approximately 100 kilobases of genomic DNA and consisting of 5592 base pairs of coding sequence contained in 22 exons. There is one large exon, exon 11, which makes up about 60% of the coding region. The 22 exons code for a protein of 1863 amino acids. This protein contains a zinc finger region close to the amino terminal which suggests that BRCA1 may be involved in regulation of gene transcription. Over 100 mutations of BRCA1 have been reported to date. Many different types of mutation are found including mis-sense and nonsense mutations, deletions, insertions and intronic mutations. A total of 70–80% of mutations of BRCA1 are frameshift mutations causing premature protein termination. BRCA1 is thought to be either a tumour suppressor gene or a gene involved in DNA repair.

Genetic alterations of BRCA1 have been identified in approximately 10% of sporadic ovarian cancers but no sporadic breast cancers. The true incidence of germline mutations in the general population remains unknown but it is estimated that between 1 in 200 and 1 in 400 women are carriers of the BRCA1 mutation. This incidence is higher in Ashkenazai Jewish women who have an incidence of about 1 in 107 of a specific frame shift mutation at position 185 in exon 2 of BRCA1 which involves deletion of adenine and guanine – 185delAG. Approximately 45% of early-onset breast cancers are considered to be linked to BRCA1. The risk of developing breast cancer in BRCA1 carriers is estimated to be between 45% and 85%. BRCA1 was previously thought not to be associated with an increased risk of male breast cancer but recently a mutation of BRCA1 has been identified in a male with breast and prostate cancer. Male carriers of BRCA1 do appear to have an increased risk of prostate cancer with an absolute risk estimated at 6–8% by 70 years of age and a relative risk of 2.9–3.3 compared with non-carriers. Both men and women with specific BRCA1 mutations also have an increased risk of colonic cancer of about 6–8% by 70 years of age which is a relative risk of between 3.3 and 4.1 compared with that of non-carriers.

A second gene BRCA2 was identified in 1994 and has been mapped to the long arm of chromosome 13. Like BRCA1, BRCA2 appears to be a tumour suppressor gene. BRCA2 codes for a protein of 2329 amino acids; the function of this protein remains unknown. Mutations of

BRCA2 may be responsible for 45% of cases of hereditary breast cancer. Families in which this abnormal gene is present show mainly a high incidence of breast cancer. Although the risk of ovarian cancer is elevated with BRCA2 mutations, the increase in risk is much lower than that seen with BRCA1 mutations. The presence of a BRCA2 mutation is also thought to be a factor in the development of certain cases of male breast cancer. The lifetime risk of developing breast cancer in a BRCA2 carrier is between 45% and 85%.

Mutation of the p53 gene on the short arm of chromosome 17 occurs in the Li-Fraumeni syndrome, a syndrome first described in 1969 and associated with early-onset bilateral breast cancer and other tumours such as soft tissue sarcomas, osteosarcomas, brain tumours, leukaemias and adrenalcortical carcinomas. Other tumours that may occur in association with this syndrome include carcinomas of the lung, prostate and pancreas, and malignant melanoma. Approximately 50% of families with Li-Fraumeni syndrome do not have germ line mutations of the p53 gene. The risk of breast cancer is over 50% by age 50 in women with this syndrome. Germ line mutations of this gene are, however, probably responsible for less than 1% of all breast cancers.

Ataxia telangiectasia is an autosomal recessive disorder in which both heterozygotes and homozygotes carrying the defective gene appear to have an increased risk of cancer, especially breast cancer. The defective gene has been mapped to a region on the long arm of chromosome 11. The coding portion of the gene consists of 100 base pairs in which over 40 mutations have so far been described. It was originally estimated that the relative risk of cancer in heterozygous females compared to that of the general population was 5.1–6.8 times that expected but recent data have questioned this. It was also thought that exposure to radiation could increase the risk of breast cancer in women who are heterozygous for the ataxia telangiectasia gene but more recent data have not confirmed radiation sensitivity. A recent study looking at patients treated for breast cancer by lumpectomy and radiotherapy showed no association between marked radiotherapy reactions and heterozygotes for the ataxia telangiectasia gene. It remains to be determined, therefore, whether radiation, including mammography, is associated with any increased risk of breast cancer in these women.

Other genes have been identified as being associated with breast cancer. This includes Cowden's disease, which is associated with a gene on chromosome 10 and is characterized by early onset of cancer, a high incidence of bilateral disease and hamartomas of the skin and the gastrointestinal tract. Gorlin's syndrome which manifest as multiple basal cell carcinomas of the skin, cysts of the jaw bones and erythematous pitting of the palms and soles is also associated with predisposition to the development of breast cancer.

Identification of women at high risk of breast cancer begins by taking an accurate family history. Between 6% and 19% of individuals with breast cancer have an affected relative, but this does not reliably identify women who are likely to be carriers of germ line mutations. In large families, a positive family history may reflect the high incidence of sporadic disease and, in small families, the absence of a family history does not rule out the presence of a genetic mutation. BRCA1 mutations may also be transmitted through male relatives in a family with no male or female breast cancers being manifest. Other individuals may exhibit *de novo* germ line mutations and consequently have no family history of breast cancer. Identification of BRCA1 carriers by family history can also be obscured by incomplete penetrance of this gene. Lifetime disease penetrance in some families is less than 50%. As this particular patient has a strong family history, she is potentially an appropriate candidate for gene testing.

Genetic tests are now available that can identify mutations of BRCA1, BRCA2 and p53 genes. There are more than a dozen laboratories carrying out BRCA1 testing within the guidelines of a protocol in the USA. Before referral for screening, some centres request that three first-degree relatives be affected, others request four. It is useful to test an unaffected relative to confirm that any mutation found in an individual is a stable abnormality. Routine genetic testing involving a sequencing of a complete BRCA1 gene is not practical. There are three common specific mutations which appear to be relatively common and these make simple diagnostic tests for these mutations possible. They are the 5382insC mutation in codon 1756, the 185delAG mutation in codon 23 and the 4184del4 mutation in codon 1355. Mutation detection after identification of affected individuals is not usually primarily by sequencing. In the absence of the three common mutations, screening for unknown mutations is carried out using techniques such as the protein truncation test and single-stranded conformational polymorphisms of chemical cleavage. Only patients in whom abnormalities are shown by these techniques have their BRCA1 gene sequenced.

Not all patients who are candidates for the procedure opt to undergo genetic testing. Testing raises the possibility of genetic discrimination and some patients will opt for clinical follow up regardless of their level of risk. Also genetic testing may not provide useful information. These issues need to be carefully considered in a genetic counselling session prior to making a decision about undergoing testing. The value of genetic testing in an unaffected individual is greatly enhanced by testing a relative with breast cancer first and demonstrating the presence of a mutation. If an affected relative is not found to have a mutation of BRCA1 or BRCA2, a negative test in an unaffected individual can occur either because she is not at an increased risk, or because there is an unidentifiable predisposing gene present in her family.

The patient decides to undergo genetic testing after her mother is found to have a BRCA1 mutation, and she is also found to have a mutation. What are the options for management?

A mutation in BRCA1 is associated with a lifetime risk of breast cancer development of between 45 to 80% and a 30–40% lifetime risk of developing ovarian carcinoma. If this level of risk is unacceptable to the patient, bilateral prophylactic mastectomies, usually with immediate breast reconstruction combined with bilateral oophorectomy, is one option. The mastectomies should be done to the same anatomic limits as a therapeutic mastectomy with removal of the nipple areolar complex to maximize the amount of breast tissue removed. Even a well-performed prophylactic mastectomy does not provide 100% protection against the development of breast cancer since small amounts of breast tissue will be left behind on the skin flaps. The level of risk in women with genetic mutations who undergo prophylactic mastectomy is not absolutely clear, although a recent large study from the Mayo Clinic demonstrated that patients who had a prophylactic subcutaneous mastectomy had a reduction of risk of approximately 90%.

For patients who do not wish surgery, ongoing studies are evaluating the role of MRI as a screening method in these young women. There are also ongoing studies evaluating the role of tamoxifen. A recent American study was halted 14 months earlier than planned when they identified a 45% reduction in the incidence of breast cancer among women who took tamoxifen compared with those who took placebo. The double-blind trial included 13,388 healthy women at high risk of developing breast cancer. In the group of women randomized to take 20 mg of tamoxifen a day, there were 85 cases of invasive breast cancer compared with 154 cases in the women assigned to the placebo group. The women were followed on average for 4 years. A summary of the results subdivided into age groups is shown in Figure 20.1. Overall, eight women died of breast cancer during the study, three in the tamoxifen cohort and five in the placebo arm. One benefit seen in postmenopausal women taking tamoxifen was a reduction in the incidence of fractures of the hip, wrist and spine; there were 47 such fractures in women taking tamoxifen compared with 71 in the placebo arm. There were 33 cases of endometrial cancer in women taking tamoxifen compared with 14 in those taking placebo. Most were early endometrial cancers, although one woman in the placebo group died of endometrial cancer. There were 17 cases of pulmonary embolus and 30 of deep vein thrombosis in the tamoxifen group compared with only 6 and 19 in the placebo group. When the study was analysed according to age, women aged under 50 seemed to be free of the adverse effects. Patients aged over 50 were at increased risk of these effects but also benefited the most from the reduction of risk of

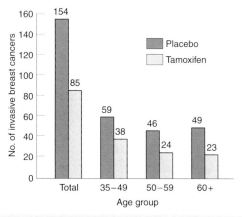

Fig. 20.1 Effect of tamoxifen on the incidence of breast cancer in the NSABP study.

breast cancer from taking tamoxifen (Figure 20.1). Raloxifene, an 'anti-oestrogen' without endometrial effects, given to women with osteoporosis has also been reported to significantly reduce breast cancer incidence. The results are not surprising as a reduction in the incidence of contralateral cancers has been demonstrated in most trials where tamoxifen is used as adjuvant therapy.

The recent Oxford Overview Analysis demonstrates the same magnitude of risk reduction in contralateral breast cancer after 5 years of tamoxifen. This benefit continues even after tamoxifen is stopped and should relieve some of the concerns that tamoxifen may only be suppressing clinically occult cancers which will regrow after tamoxifen is stopped. We also do not know if tamoxifen is equally effective in preventing breast cancer in all risk groups. Women at risk due to atypical hyperplasia and lobular carcinoma *in situ* had clear benefit in the NSABP trial. No specific data is available for women at risk on the basis of genetic mutation. There is some evidence that certain women at very high risk of breast cancer, such as BRCA1 germ line mutation carriers, are predisposed to develop hormone-independent tumours which are less likely to be affected by the preventive action of tamoxifen. There is some controversy about the current role of tamoxifen for prevention since a small British study of high risk women and an Italian trial of women at average risk failed to demonstrate a reduction in breast cancer incidence with tamoxifen. Both of these studies had significantly less power than the NSABP study, due to small sample size or low breast cancer incidence. The Food and Drug Administration has approved tamoxifen for prevention, and for many women it is a welcome alternative to prophylactic mastectomy or a watch and wait policy.

An alternative to prophylactic surgery or anti-oestrogen therapy is close clinical surveillance, which consists of instruction in breast self-examination, twice yearly breast examinations by a health care provider and an annual screening mammogram. This strategy is designed to detect cancer at an early stage should it develop, and obviously does nothing to reduce risk. The algorithm for evaluation and management of the woman at increased risk for breast cancer is summarized in Figure 20.2.

1. Assess risk factors
   Family history → genetic counselling
   Reproductive history
   Age
   Prior breast cancer
   Radiation exposure
   High-risk benign breast pathology → second opinion

2. Identify competing causes of mortality

3. Clinical evaluation
   Breast examination – evaluate difficulty
   Mammogram – adequacy of visualization

4. Discuss with patient

Patient choice

Observation
Monthly breast self-examination
Annual mammography
Clinical examination 4–6 months
Research trial
Tamoxifen 20 mg qd x 5 years

Prophylactic mastectomy
Consultation regarding reconstruction
Psychological evaluation

Fig. 20.2 Evaluation and management of a woman at increased risk of breast cancer.

The patient opts for careful surveillance and 3 years later is found to have a 1 cm, grade 2 infiltrating ductal carcinoma. Does her genetic status affect her local therapy options?

Limited information is available on the impact of genetic mutation on the outcome of local therapy. A single study examining mastectomy specimens in patients with genetic mutations has not identified a higher incidence of multicentricity or multifocality which would be a contraindication to breast conserving therapy. In the patient who opts for mastectomy with a TRAM flap reconstruction as primary therapy, the increased risk of contralateral primary breast carcinoma and the inability to perform a second TRAM procedure should prompt a discussion of the pros and cons of contralateral prophylactic mastectomy at the time of the initial surgery. Likewise, in a patient with a very small breast who opts for a reconstruction using tissue expansion, the pros and cons of gaining symmetry by performing a contralateral prophylactic mastectomy should be discussed.

21 A 50-year-old woman with microcalcification on mammography

M Morrow

A 50-year-old woman whose mother had breast cancer at age 65 has a mammogram which demonstrates a cluster of microcalcifications in the right breast. Biopsy of the area demonstrates atypical ductal hyperplasia. What is the appropriate management of this lesion?

Atypical ductal hyperplasia is a risk factor for breast cancer development. In the absence of a family history of breast cancer, only about 10% of women with this diagnosis will develop carcinoma in a 10-year period (relative risk 4–5) (Table 21.1). The combination of atypical hyperplasia and a first-degree relative with breast cancer increases the relative risk to 9, or approximately 20% over 10 years (Figure 21.1). Close surveillance of these women with annual mammography and twice-yearly physician examination is standard treatment. A baseline mammogram of the right breast 6 months after biopsy will confirm complete excision of the calcifications and document the appearance of the biopsy scar for comparison with future studies.

Table 21.1 Risk of developing breast cancer associated with risk factors

Factors present	Approximate risk
Atypical hyperplasia (specifically defined)	10–15% in next 15–20 years
Atypical hyperplasia and family history of breast cancer*	20–30% in next 15–20 years
Carrier of mutant BRCA1 gene	60–85% during lifetime

*Disease in first-degree relative (mother, sister or daughter).

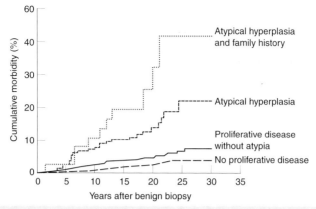

Fig. 21.1 Risk of subsequent development of invasive carcinoma in patients with no epithelial proliferation, proliferative disease without atypia (moderate or florid hyperplasia), atypical hyperplasia, or atypical hyperplasia and a family history of cancer. (From: Dixon JM. ABC of Breast Diseases. London: BMJ Publishing Group 1995; p. 63, with permission.)

What are the other risk factors for breast cancer?

The most obvious risk factor is age. The incidence of breast cancer increases with age, doubling about every 10 years until the menopause, when the rate of increase slows dramatically. In some countries there is a flattening of the age incidence curve after the menopause (Figure 21.2). In Western countries, approximately 50% of the lifetime risk of breast cancer is seen after the age of 65.

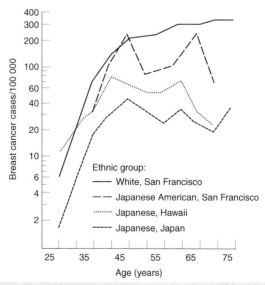

Fig. 21.2 Annual incidence of breast cancer in Japanese women in Japan, Hawaii and San Francisco and in white women from San Francisco. (From: Dixon JM. ABC of Breast Diseases. London: BMJ Publishing Group 1995; p. 19, with permission.)

There is a marked geographic variation in the age-adjusted incidence of breast cancer that varies approximately five times between different countries. The difference is most marked between Far Eastern and Western countries. Studies of migrants from Japan to Hawaii show that the rates of breast cancer in migrants assume the rate in the host country within one to two generations, indicating that environmental factors are more important than genetic factors in the aetiology of breast cancer.

Women who start menstruating early in life or who have a late menopause are at an increased risk of developing breast cancer. Women who have a natural menopause after the age of 55 are twice as likely to develop breast cancer as women who experience the menopause before the age of 45. At one extreme, women who undergo bilateral oophorectomy before the age of 35 have only 40% the risk of breast cancer of women who have a natural menopause.

Nulliparity and late age at first birth both increase lifetime risk of breast cancer. For a women who has her first child after the age of 30, her risk is about twice that of a woman who has her first child before the age of 20. The highest risk group is those who have their first child after the age of 35 with these women being at even higher risk than those women who have no children at all.

Apart from women with severe atypical epithelial hyperplasia, women with palpable cysts, complex fibroadenomas, duct papillomas, sclerosing adenosis and moderate or florid epithelial hyperplasia have a slightly higher risk of breast cancer (1.5–3 times) than women without these changes, but a relative risk of less than four is deemed not clinically significant (Table 21.2).

A doubling of the risk of breast cancer later in life was observed among teenage girls exposed to radiation during the Second World War. Ionizing radiation also increases risk later in life, particularly when exposure is during the period of rapid breast development. Mammographic screening is associated with a net decrease in mortality from breast cancer in women over the age of 50. It has been calculated that, for every 2 million women aged over 50 who have been screened by means of a single mammogram, one extra cancer a year after 10 years may be caused by the radiation delivered to the breast. Compared with an incidence of breast cancer, which approaches 2000 every million women aged 60, the risk of causing

Table 21.2 Relative risk of invasive breast cancer associated with benign diseases

No increased risk
  Mild hyperplasia
  Duct ectasia
  Apocrine metaplasia
  Simple fibroadenomas
  Microcysts
  Periductal mastitis
  Adenosis

Slightly increased risk (1.5–2 times)
  Moderate and florid hyperplasia
  Papilloma
  Complex fibroadenomas
  Sclerosing adenosis
  Palpable breast cysts*

Moderately increased risk (4–5 times)
  Atypical hyperplasia

*Palpable breast cysts are probably associated with a relative risk in the order of two to three times that of the general population.

breast cancer compared with the chances of detecting the disease are very small.

Although there is a close correlation between the incidence of breast cancer and dietary fat intake in populations, the true relationship between fat intake and breast cancer does not appear to be particularly strong or consistent. Obesity is associated with a twofold increase in the risk of breast cancer in post-menopausal women. Some studies have shown a link between alcohol consumption and the incidence of breast cancer but the relationship is inconsistent.

While women are taking the oral contraceptive agent they have a small increase in the relative risk of developing breast cancer of 1.24 times that of age-matched controls. One to four years after stopping the oral contraceptive pill the risk is 1.16 and 5–9 years after stopping the risk is 1.07. There is no significant excess risk of having breast cancer diagnosed 10 or more years after stopping use of the pill and the oral contraceptive does not increase the risk of the more common post-menopausal breast cancer. The cancers diagnosed in women who have used oral contraceptives appear less clinically advanced than those diagnosed in women who have never used the pill. Although women who begin use of the pill before the age of 20 have a higher

Table 21.3 Relationship of hormone replacement therapy (HRT) to breast cancer development

Time on HRT	Breast cancers over the 20 years from age 50–70	Extra breast cancers in HRT users	Individual risk of women over 20 years
Never	45 per 1000	—	1 in 22
5 years' use	47 per 1000	2 per 1000	1 in 21
10 years' use	51 per 1000	6 per 1000	1 in 19
15 years' use	57 per 1000	12 per 1000	1 in 17–18

relative risk of having breast cancer diagnosed while they are taking the oral contraceptive pill than older women, these relative risks apply at an age when breast cancer is rare. The relationship of hormone replacement therapy and breast cancer is somewhat similar in that there is an increased risk of breast cancer in women while they are taking HRT (Table 21.3). The risk increases as length of time on hormone replacement therapy increases and only becomes clinically significant after 10 years. The risks associated with HRT disappear 5 years after stopping this treatment.

The patient is perimenopausal and has severe hot flushes, and mood swings. Is hormone replacement appropriate?

The risks associated with hormone replacement therapy are outlined above. In the subset of women at increased risk whether due to family history of breast cancer or atypical hyperplasia, HRT has not been shown to have different effects from that in the general population. The greatest concern is with long-term high-dose HRT. One approach to this patient would be to treat her with HRT for a brief (1–3 years) period around the menopause for symptom relief. In the woman with an intact uterus, a combination of oestrogen and progesterone is indicated to avoid the increased incidence of endometrial carcinoma seen with the use of unopposed oestrogen. The long-term benefits of HRT, including protection against osteoporosis and cardiac disease can be obtained with other non-hormonal agents after menopausal symptoms have been relieved. The new selective oestrogen receptor modulating drugs (e.g. raloxifene) are particularly attractive in this regard. Progesterone preparations alone have been reported to reduce the incidence and severity of hot flushes (e.g. megestrol acetate 20 mg BD). However, they have stimulatory effects on breast cells which are similar to those seen with oestrogen, and cannot be assumed to have no effect on breast cancer risk.

Non-hormonal alternatives for hot flushes include bellergal and clonidine. Neither of these are particularly effective, and both have a significant incidence of side effects. Herbal preparations have become very popular for the treatment of perimenopausal symptoms and may be effective because many of them contain phyto-oestrogens.

Two years later, a new cluster of microcalcification develops in the opposite breast. Biopsy reveals a 1.5 cm high-grade ductal carcinoma *in situ* (DCIS). What do we know about the natural history of DCIS?

Carcinoma cells confined to within the terminal duct lobular unit and the adjacent ducts but which have not yet invaded through the basement membrane are known as carcinoma *in situ*. As with invasive disease, two main types have been described; ductal carcinoma *in situ* and lobular carcinoma *in situ* (LCIS). DCIS has a variety of presentations. It may present as a palpable mass, although only 1–2% of palpable carcinomas are DCIS, or it may present as nipple discharge or Paget's disease of the nipple. Today, mammographically detected DCIS is the most frequent presentation. The majority of DCIS presents as microcalcification. Linear, ductal-type calcifications are characteristically seen with comedo DCIS (Figure 21.3) while cribriform and micropapillary DCIS often have finer sand-like calcifications. While LCIS tends to occur in its pure form, DCIS often

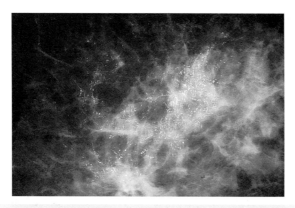

Fig. 21.3 Comedo ductal carcinoma *in situ*.

occurs as a mixture of different types: comedo, cribriform, micropapillary and solid. For this reason a variety of classification systems have been developed to try to group different types of DCIS with similar biologic potential. These classifications generally combine grade and the presence or absence of necrosis. As yet, none have been prospectively shown to predict the behaviour of DCIS.

Many more patients with DCIS are now being diagnosed as the national breast screening programmes become fully operational. Prior to the institution of breast screening, DCIS was uncommon and accounted for 5% or less of malignancies but, with the advent of screening, there has been a surprising increase in the frequency, particularly over the last decade. In 1993 there were an estimated 4900 cases of DCIS in the USA but a decade later the number had increased to over 23,000. This increase has been across all age groups, with a 12% annual increase in the 40–49 year age group and a 15.1% annual increase in women over the age of 50. This increase appears to be real, and it does not represent overdiagnosis. There are some ground rules, and a lesion measuring < 3 mm in size is more likely to be atypical ductal hyperplasia (ADH) than DCIS and should be diagnosed as such. There are some ADH lesions which are larger, but lesions over 6 mm are rarely examples of ADH. There is considerable consistency in large and high/intermediate-grade lesions which constitute the majority of cases of DCIS.

Reports of the natural history of DCIS are based on a review of biopsies performed many years earlier which were classified by the original pathologist as benign, a few of which on subsequent review were recognized as having areas of DCIS. A recently updated study from Nashville of 28 patients with DCIS undiagnosed on biopsy reports that by 30 years 40% had developed an invasive breast cancer, all at the site of the original biopsy. The 40% who developed breast cancer were thought to belong to the group where it was considered that the biopsy did not remove all the DCIS. A second study from New York reported similar rates of cancer development. All lesions in the Nashville and New York series were low grade. A third study of 80 patients included two patients with high-grade DCIS and significant numbers of patients with lesions that others call ADH. After a mean follow up of 17.5 years, 20% of women in this series had developed invasive cancer or recurrent DCIS. From these data it appears that, following an incomplete excision, between 20% and 60% of patients with low-grade DCIS will develop recurrent DCIS or an invasive cancer at the same site in the breast over a 20-year period, with the majority of these developing within the first decade. There is little information on the behaviour of inadequately excised intermediate and high-grade DCIS, although there is the suspicion that recurrence may occur more often. It is exemplified by an 80% recurrence rate at 5 years reported in one series in patients with high-grade DCIS treated by wide excision alone.

Treating all DCIS lesions in the same manner makes little sense as studies have shown marked biological and behavioural differences between different histological types of DCIS. Biological differences include difference in oncogene expression, with 80% of high-grade DCIS staining positive for the oncogene erbB2 whereas only 10% of low-grade DCIS expresses erbB2; the same is true for the tumour suppressor gene p53 with over 60% of high-grade but less than 5% of low-grade lesions demonstrating overexpression. The presence of significant amounts of oestrogen receptor (ER) also differs between different histological subtypes with 28% of comedo DCIS being ER-positive compared with 50% in non-comedo DCIS.

What are the management options for this patient?

Management options for DCIS include total mastectomy, excision alone and excision and irradiation (XRT). Treatment with excision and XRT has a risk of recurrence of 10–15% over 10 years and half of the recurrences are invasive carcinoma. The cause-specific mortality at 10 years is approximately 3%. It was initially thought that breast recurrences were more frequent after treatment of high-grade DCIS with excision and XRT than when the same treatment was used for low- and intermediate-grade DCIS. In fact, local failures tend to occur earlier with high-grade lesions, so studies with short follow up will underestimate the risk of recurrence in low-grade lesions. At 10 years, the risk of recurrence is equal for the two groups. Non-randomized studies of highly selected patients with DCIS treated by excision alone, which include usually those with small, low-grade lesions, demonstrate local failure rates similar to those seen with excision and XRT. An update of the only published randomized trial comparing these two treatments, (Table 21.4), NSABP B17, demonstrated that XRT reduced the risk of invasive carcinoma by

Table 21.4 Results of the National Surgical Adjuvant Breast Project (NSABP) DCIS Trial (B-17) with a median follow up of 8 years

Treatment	Number of women	% with recurrent		Total % recurrence
		DCIS	Invasive cancer	
Wide excision	403	13	13	26
Wide excision + radiotherapy	411	7	4	11

approximately 69% and the risk of recurrent DCIS by 42%. After a mean follow up of 8 years, 26% of the patients treated by wide local excision alone developed local recurrence. Since an invasive local failure has the potential to increase breast cancer mortality, there has been great interest in identifying predictive factors for treatment selection. The Van Nuys index combines tumour size, grade and margin width to select treatment. It is important to recognize that the tissue-processing techniques essential to the derivation of this index are not universally in use. A number of other methodologic problems are present, the most important of which is that the index requires prospective confirmation. In addition, the role of other variables such as age and family history, which are not included in the index, require evaluation.

The full pathology report on this patient indicates that the DCIS is high grade, has marked necrosis with calcification and the tumour has been completely excised with a minimum 5 mm margin. How should she be treated?

According to the Van Nuys prognostic index, this lesion has a score of 3 on pathology, 2 on margin of excision and 1 extent, giving a total score of 6. This falls into the category of patients who would benefit from radiotherapy. In patients with microcalcifications, a post-excision mammogram to document complete removal of all microcalcifications is performed prior to beginning XRT.

If the pathology had demonstrated disease at the excision margins, what would have been the options for this patient?

The first option would have been re-excision. By orientating the initial specimen when it was submitted to the pathologist it should be possible to obtain information on exactly which of the lateral margins is involved and re-excision can then be limited to removing tissue from the involved margin. A second option is to proceed to mastectomy with or without immediate breast reconstruction. This option is more appropriate in patients who have had a large initial excision relative to the size of the breast and in patients who have multiple involved margins.

A re-excision is performed and this shows extensive DCIS extending to the new margins of resection. What is the appropriate management?

The feasibility of a further attempt at breast conservation depends on the size of the patient's breast and the ability to perform a cosmetically satisfactory re-excision. This can be attempted with the understanding that the inability to obtain a tumour-free margin will necessitate a subsequent mastectomy. Total or simple mastectomy, with or without immediate breast reconstruction, is the option most clinicians used for this patient. Recurrence rates after mastectomy are less than 2%, regardless of the size or grade of DCIS. Axillary dissection is not indicated in the management of DCIS since nodal metastases are present in fewer than 3% of patients. Management options for patients with DCIS are summarized in Figure 21.4. Patients undergoing mastectomy can have skin sparing mastectomy. It is usual to remove

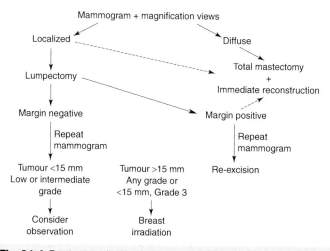

Fig. 21.4 Treatment selection in the patient with DCIS.

the nipple. An incision just outside the areola removes the nipple/ areola complex and allows a complete mastectomy to be performed. Immediate reconstruction either with a latissimus dorsi flap and implant or a TRAM flap is then possible.

Does this patient require adjuvant systemic therapy?

The purpose of adjuvant therapy is to reduce the risk of distant metastases, which by definition do not occur in DCIS. Predictors of the risk of metastases in invasive carcinoma such as tumour size or grade do not have the same implications in DCIS. There is no indication for adjuvant chemotherapy or tamoxifen in a patient with DCIS. The role of tamoxifen in reducing local recurrence after breast preservation in DCIS is under study.

A 42-year-old premenopausal woman with a painless right breast lump

W Gradishar, M Morrow, D Watson and J M Dixon

Mrs Jones is a 42-year-old premenopausal woman who presents with a 6-week history of a painless right breast lump which has persisted through one menstrual cycle. On clinical examination she has a 1.3 cm mass in the upper outer quadrant of the right breast, with no associated skin or nipple changes, and no palpable axillary or supraclavicular adenopathy. What investigations would you perform to establish the diagnosis?

The diagnostic investigation in this patient is fine-needle aspiration. If the mass is a cyst, this procedure will be both diagnostic and therapeutic. If the mass is solid, cellular material can be obtained for diagnosis. In addition, bilateral mammography with spot compression views of the mass will be valuable particularly if the mass is solid. The purpose of the mammogram is not to determine the necessity for a biopsy, but to document the extent of the lesion and identify any clinically occult multicentric disease in the ipsilateral breast or additional lesions in the contralateral breast. Ultrasonography can provide valuable information on whether a lesion is solid or cystic (see Figure 13.6), and it provides a very accurate assessment of the size of a malignant mass lesion. The characteristic features on ultrasound are an irregular mass with acoustic shadowing behind (Figure 22.1). If an unequivocal diagnosis of malignancy is made on cytology and this is supported by findings on clinical examination and on imaging, then it is appropriate to proceed to definitive local therapy. A 14 gauge core needle biopsy performed using an automatic gun is an alternative outpatient procedure to establish the diagnosis of solid breast masses, particularly when a qualified cytopathologist is not available. It is also of value where an unequivocal diagnosis cannot be obtained by

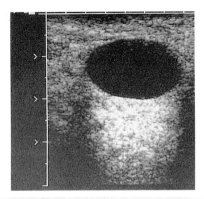

Fig. 22.1 Cyst on ultrasound.

cytology. Diagnostic accuracy with the new automatic core biopsy guns is only slightly less than that obtained with fine-needle aspiration cytology (Table 13.1). It is performed after infiltration of local anaesthesia. It can be uncomfortable but, providing sufficient local anaesthetic is used (1% lignocaine or lidocaine with 1:200,000 adrenaline), the procedure should not be painful. Diagnostic biopsy should be reserved for patients where a definitive diagnosis cannot be established by needle biopsy techniques.

If cancer is confirmed, what other investigations are necessary?

Additional investigations in this patient should be directed toward identifying metastases which could alter the treatment plan. In this clinical stage 1 carcinoma, the risk of metastatic disease is low. This patient should have blood taken for a full blood count, tests of liver function, serum calcium and alkaline phosphatase, and possibly also a chest X-ray. Some centres now restrict routine chest radiographs to patients over the age of 50. Bone and liver scans in a patient with such a small lesion should not be performed unless the patient has localized specific symptoms.

What are the options for local therapy in this patient?

This patient is a candidate for breast conserving therapy consisting of a wide local excision, combined with some form of axillary surgery and breast irradiation or a modified radical mastectomy alone, with or without immediate breast reconstruction. Survival after breast-conserving therapy and mastectomy does not differ. Criteria for

Table 22.1 Indications and contraindications for selection of patients for breast conservation (adapted from NIH Consensus Conference Statement, 1991)

Indications	T1, T2 ($\leqslant$ 4 cm), N0, N1, M0
	T2 > 4 cm in large breasts
Contraindications	T3–4, N2, M1
	Large or central tumours in small breasts
	Multifocal/multicentric disease
	Collagen vascular disease
	Prior irradiation of the breast region
	Pregnancy

selection for treatment by breast conservation is outlined in Table 22.1. When medically equivalent treatment options are available, these should be discussed with the patient, and the role and extent of the patient's wishes to be involved in decision making ascertained. The contraindications to breast-conserving therapy are a history of prior breast irradiation, pregnancy, multicentric or extensive multifocal disease, and the presence of scleroderma or lupus.

Breast conservation is usually restricted to carcinomas less than 4 cm, although it may not be appropriate to perform breast conservation in smaller cancers in small breasts. Conversely, for patients with larger breasts, breast conservation for tumours larger than 5 cm may result in an acceptable cosmetic outcome. None of these factors are present in this case and only about 10% of patients with clinical stage 1 carcinoma have contraindications to breast-conserving therapy. Should mastectomy be indicated or selected by the patient, the only contraindication to immediate breast reconstruction is the presence of co-morbid conditions which would make prolongation of general anaesthesia unwise.

There is controversy as to the extent to which the axilla should be dissected in patients with operable breast cancer. Approximately 75% of the lymph from the breast drains to the axilla, with the remainder going to the internal mammary nodes. Axillary lymph node status remains the single most important prognostic factor. The greater the number of nodes involved, the worse the prognosis (Figure 22.2) with an average 10-year survival of 60–70% for node-negative patients dropping to 20–30% for those with involved nodes, in the absence of adjuvant therapy.

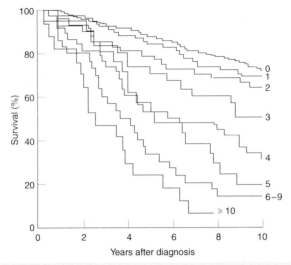

Fig. 22.2 Number of nodes involved in relation to survival. (From: Dixon JM. ABC of Breast Diseases. London: BMJ Publishing Group 1995; p. 31, with permission.)

The axillary contents can be divided into three levels (Figure 22.3). The level I nodes are those inferior and lateral to the pectoralis minor, the level II nodes are posterior to the pectoralis minor and inferior to the axillary vein, and the level III nodes are below the axillary vein and medial to the pectoralis minor. There is agreement that isolated metastases to level III nodes are very infrequent, occurring in less than 2% of patients. This is not surprising since the mean number of nodes in level III is 2-3. Reports of the likelihood of metastases at level II in

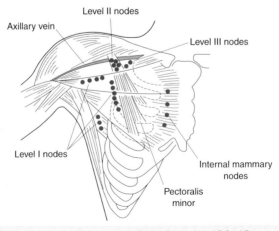

Fig. 22.3 Levels of axillary nodes. (From: Dixon JM. ABC of Breast Diseases. London: BMJ Publishing Group 1995; p. 30, with permission.)

the absence of disease at level I, so called 'skip metastases' are more variable. Isolated metastases to level II are reported in as many as 20% of patients in some studies. This has led to the recommendation in the USA that a level I and II dissection should be performed to ensure adequate axillary staging, with level III dissections reserved for patients who have evidence of gross nodal involvement at the time of surgery. Although concern has been expressed that a two-level dissection will leave behind nodal metastases in some patients, axillary recurrences are seen in only 2–3% of such patients. The common practice of irradiating a supraclavicular field (which includes the axillary apex) when four or more nodes are found to contain metastases also minimizes the risk of axillary failure. Studies which have examined the risk of axillary failure in node negative axillary dissections on the basis of the number of nodes removed have shown that the removal of 10 or more nodes is associated with a very low incidence of axillary recurrence.

More controversy has surrounded the use of axillary sampling procedures. These operations are much less well defined. Some centres have shown that they can consistently stage the axilla with the removal of a limited number of nodes, while others have been unable to reproduce these results.

Recently, sentinel node biopsy has been proposed as an alternative to the use of axillary dissection for some patients. Sentinel node biopsy is performed by injecting isosulfan blue or Tc-labelled sulphur colloid or albumin either subdermally directly over the primary tumour site or into the breast tissue around the tumour and either visually identifying the blue node in the axilla, or using a hand-held probe to detect the radioactive node. Several studies using blue dye alone, radioactivity alone, or a combination of the two techniques have shown that a sentinel node can be identified in 90% of patients and that it will accurately predict the status of the remaining axillary nodes in greater than 95% of cases. Axillary dissection is then limited to patients with involvement of the sentinel node. When frozen section is used to assess the status of the sentinel node, approximately 10% of patients thought to be node negative will have tumour cells identified during complete histological assessment and will require a second operation. The sentinel node biopsy appears to allow accurate axillary staging while minimizing morbidity but requires further evaluation before being introduced into routine practice. Furthermore, additional information on the accuracy of the technique for large tumours, multifocal tumours, patients with large biopsy cavities, and previous surgery is needed before this becomes the standard of care for all patients.

Axillary surgery has complications with include lymphoedema, damage to the nerves in the axilla (surgically this is division of the intercostobrachial, long thoracic or thoracodorsal nerves) and with radiotherapy there is the rare complication of brachial plexopathy. One study of axillary surgery reported that 70% of patients following axillary surgery complained of numbness, 33% of pain, 25% of weakness, 24% of limb swelling and 15% of arm stiffness. Objectively, at 4 years after surgery, numbness was present in 55%, weakness in 27%, limb swelling in 15% and stiffness in 12%. In this study, 39% of patients indicated that axillary clearance had had some effect on their lives. A complete axillary clearance to level III is therefore not without morbidity. Even greater morbidity follows the combination of extensive axillary surgery and radiotherapy with lymphoedema rates of over 40%. Brachial plexopathy is due in part to overlapping of radiotherapy fields which can result in high doses of radiation being delivered to the brachial plexus. With modern planning techniques and treatment schedules and new equipment, this complication is rare. Both surgery and radiotherapy are associated with a reduction in the range of movement of the shoulder in some patients and about 5% of patients develop a frozen shoulder. This can be minimized by regular exercise programmes developed and supervised by a physiotherapist.

What factors affect cosmetic outcome after breast conservation?

Although a variety of factors have been shown to influence cosmesis, the amount of breast tissue which is excised is the major determinant of cosmetic outcome. Attempting to reapproximate the breast tissue can result in changes in breast contour which may not be visible with the patient in the supine position. The extent of breast resection which is needed to optimize local control will vary with the characteristics of the primary tumour, but in general, excision of the tumour with a small margin of grossly normal breast tissue (approximately 1 cm) should be the initial procedure. Skin removal is not necessary or desirable since it often alters the position of the nipple. Skin excision should be reserved for superficial tumours where the lesion abuts the dermis. Other factors which have been reported to

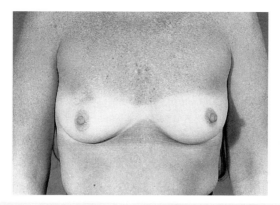

Fig. 22.4 Good cosmesis after breast conservation.

influence cosmesis include very large breast size, the extent of axillary surgery, the use of radiotherapy boost to the tumour bed, and the experience of the treating physicians.

Overall, approximately 90% of patients rate their cosmetic outcome as good or excellent (Figure 22.4) after the completion of therapy, but 10% have a poor result (Figure 22.5). The final cosmetic appearance of the breast is usually evident three years after the completion of radiotherapy. By this time, maximum resolution of breast oedema has occurred and fibrosis and retraction, the main determinants of late cosmetic outcome, are present. After three years the appearance of the treated breast is stable, but changes in the untreated breast such as increasing ptosis due to ageing may increase the asymmetry between the treated and untreated breast.

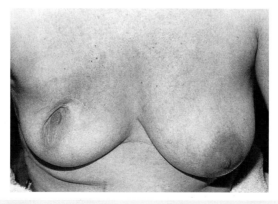

Fig. 22.5 Poor cosmesis after breast conservation.

The patient undergoes lumpectomy and has an axillary dissection to level II. Pathology demonstrates a 1.4 cm grade 2 infiltrating ductal carcinoma and an extensive intraductal component. No lymphatic/ vascular invasion is noted and the margins are negative. Zero of 18 axillary nodes contain metastases. Oestrogen and progesterone receptors are positive. With this information, is the patient suitable for treatment by breast conservation? Has she any factors which might increase her risk of local recurrence after breast conservation?

The local recurrence rates seen today after breast conservation are considerably lower than those reported 10–15 years ago, and average 6–8% at 10 years. These reductions are due to improvements in breast imaging allowing more appropriate patient selection, as well as improvements in the extent of pathologic examination of specimens and the routine use of inked margins to assess the completeness of tumour excision. In addition, treatment factors such as the increased use of adjuvant systemic therapy have also decreased local failure rates.

The presence of an extensive intraductal component (EIC), defined as being present when 25% of the primary tumour is composed of ductal carcinoma *in situ* (DCIS) and DCIS is present in the surrounding breast tissue, was initially thought to be a significant risk factor for local failure after breast conservation. This finding was primarily noted in studies where microscopic margins of resection were not assessed. More recent studies have shown that, when clear margins are obtained, patients with EIC-positive tumours have local failure rates similar to those seen in EIC-negative tumours (Table 22.2), so the finding of an EIC is not considered a contraindication to breast conservation providing that clear margins are obtained. The presence of tumour in vascular or lymphatic spaces within the breast is associated with a doubling of the risk of local recurrence after breast conservation but is also associated with an increased risk of local failure after mastectomy. Tumour size, nodal status and hormone receptor status are not predictors of the risk of breast recurrence.

Among treatment-related factors, completeness of excision is the major determinant of the risk of local recurrence. Gross or extensive microscopic tumour at the margin is associated with a 4–5-fold increase in the risk of local recurrence compared to clear margins. The

Table 22.2 Margins and extensive *in situ* component*

| | % Local recurrence | | | |
| | Boston | | Stanford | |
Margins	EIC +ve	EIC −ve	EIC +ve	EIC −ve
Positive/non-negative	37	7	21	11
Close	0	5		
Negative	0	2	0	1

*Percentage local recurrence rates in two American centres in a series of patients treated by breast conservation (wide excision and radiotherapy) subdivided on the presence or absence of an extensive *in situ* component (EIC) within the invasive cancer.

significance of a single area of microscopic tumour at the margin is uncertain, although some studies suggest that this increases the risk of late local recurrence at the primary tumour site.

Patient-related factors such as age and a family history of breast carcinoma have been suggested to influence local failure rates (Table 22.3). Although an assessment of the influence of age is complicated by a higher incidence in young women of pathologic factors such as EIC and lymphatic invasion which are known to impact upon local recurrence, after correction for these factors, women under age 35 appear to have a twofold increase in the risk of local recurrence. However, young women also have an increased risk of local failure after mastectomy compared to their older counterparts, so age is not useful for treatment selection. In contrast to age, a family history of a first- or second-degree relative with breast cancer does not influence the risk of local failure. The impact of a mutation in a breast-cancer predisposition gene on local failure is unknown at this time.

Table 22.3 Age and local recurrence

Age (years)	Local recurrence rates (%)
<35	17
35–50	12
>51	6

Table 22.4 Histological classification of breast cancer and frequency of presentation in a symptomatic population

History	% frequency
Non-invasive	
Ductal carcinoma *in situ*	6
Lobular carcinoma *in situ*	0.2
Invasive	
No special type, 'ductal carcinoma'	68
Special types	
Lobular	
Classical	3
Variants	7
Tubular	3
Cribriform	3
Medullary	3
Mucinous	2
Microinvasive	2
Papillary	1
Other rare types*	1.8

*Includes a few pure apocrine cancers, metaplastic cancers and adenodcystic cancers.

Tumours are classified into different histological types. The most common classification of invasive breast cancers separates cancers into ductal and lobular types. This classification was based on the belief that ductal carcinomas arise from ducts and lobular carcinomas from lobules. We now know that invasive ductal and lobular carcinomas both arise from the terminal duct lobular unit and this terminology is no longer appropriate, although it is still commonly used. Some so-called invasive ductal carcinomas have distinct patterns of growth and cellular morphology and, on this basis, certain types of breast cancer can be identified (Table 22.4). Those with special features are called invasive cancers of special type while the remainder are considered invasive (ductal) carcinomas of no special type. This classification has clinical relevance in that certain special type tumours have a much better prognosis than tumours that are of no special type.

Among the cancers of no special type, prognostic information can be obtained by grading the degree of differentiation of the tumour. Degrees of glandular formation, nuclear pleomorphism and frequency of mitosis is scored from 1 to 3. For example, a tumour with many glands would score 1, whereas a tumour with no glands would score 3. These values are combined and converted into three groups: grade 1 (score 3–5), grade 2 (scores 6 and 7) and grade 3 (scores 8 and 9). This derived histological grade – often known as the Bloom and Richardson grade or the Scarf, Bloom and Richardson grade after the originators of this system – is an important predictor of both local recurrence and overall survival. Patients with low-grade tumours appear to be at low risk of local recurrence following either breast conservation or mastectomy. There appears to be a stepwise increase in local recurrence as the grade increases, although not all studies have shown major differences in local recurrence rates between histological grade 2 and grade 3 cancers. There is no difference in the rates of local recurrence following breast conserving treatment between invasive carcinomas of no special type and invasive lobular carcinomas. Invasive lobular carcinomas are, however, frequently more difficult to excise completely and more likely to have involved margins.

As this patient has had a complete excision and does not have any other significant risk factors for local recurrence, she is suitable to continue with breast conservation therapy. Breast conservation therapy consists of an adequate wide local excision and whole breast radiotherapy. Lumpectomy without breast irradiation has an unacceptably high rate of local recurrence in the breast (up to 40%) and this is reduced to less than 10% by the addition of radiotherapy to the breast.

Doses of 40–50 Gy are delivered in daily fractions over 3–5 weeks. A top up or booster 10–20 Gy can be given to the excision site either by external beam irradiation or by means of radioactive implants, although it is not yet clear whether a boost is necessary.

If the pathology had demonstrated disease at the excision margins, what would have been the options for this patient?

The first option would have been re-excision. By orientating the initial specimen when it was submitted to the pathologist, it should be possible to obtain information on exactly which of the lateral margins are involved and re-excision can then be limited to removing tissue from the involved margin. A second option is to proceed to mastectomy with or without immediate breast reconstruction. This option is more appropriate in patients who have had a large initial excision relative to the size of the breast and in patients who have multiple involved margins.

Having decided to treat her with breast conservation therapy, does this patient need adjuvant systemic therapy?

This patient has a T1c, N0 stage I invasive breast cancer (Tables 22.5a and b). An estimate based on the tumour size and grade is that she has a 5-year recurrence rate of 13% and a 5-year overall survival rate of between 93% and 95%.

Predictors of survival in node-negative patients include tumour size and histological grade. There is a stepwise reduction in survival as the size of the tumour increases (Figure 22.6). Likewise, as the grade of the tumour increases, so the survival decreases (Figure 22.7).

Table 22.5a TNM staging for breast cancer

Primary tumour (T):
 TX: Primary tumour cannot be assessed
 T0: No evidence of primary tumour
 T1s: Carcinoma *in situ*; intraductal carcinoma, lobular carcinoma *in situ*, or Paget's disease of the nipple with no associated tumour mass*
 T1: Tumour 2.0 cm or less in greatest dimension†
  T1a: 0.5 cm or less in greatest dimension
  T1b: More than 0.5 cm but not more than 1.0 cm in greatest dimension
  T1c: More than 1.0 cm but not more than 2.0 cm in greatest dimension
 T2: Tumour more than 2.0 cm but not more than 5.0 cm in greatest dimension†
 T3: Tumour more than 5.0 cm in greatest dimension†
 T4: Tumour of any size with direct extension to chest wall or skin
  T4a: Extension to chest wall
  T4b: Oedema (including *peau d'orange*), ulceration of the skin of the breast or satellite nodules confined to the same breast
  T4c: Both of the above (T4a and T4b)
  T4d: Inflammatory carcinoma

Regional lymph nodes (N):
 NX: Regional lymph nodes cannot be assessed (e.g. previously removed)
 N0: No regional lymph node metastasis
 N1: Metastasis to movable ipsilateral axillary lymph node(s)
 N2: Metastasis to ipsilateral lymph node(s) fixed to one another or to other structures
 N3: Metastasis to ipsilateral internal mammary lymph node(s)

Distant metastasis (M):
 MX: Presence of distant metastasis cannot be assessed
 M0: No distant metastasis
 M1: Distant metastasis present (includes metastasis to ipsilateral supraclavicular lymph nodes)

Note: Chest wall includes ribs, intercostal muscles, and serratus anterior muscle but not pectoral muscle.
*Paget's disease associated with tumour mass is classified according to the size of the tumour.
†Dimpling of the skin, nipple retraction or other skin changes may occur in T1, T2, or T3 without changing the classification.

Table 22.5b UICC stage groupings

Stage	TNM grouping
0	Tis, N0, M0
I	T1, N0, M0
IIA	T0, N1, M0 T1, N1, M0 T2, N0, M0
IIB	T2, N1, M0 T3, N0, M0
IIIA	T0, N2, M0 T1, N2, M0 T2, N2, M0 T3, N1, M0 T3, N2, M0
IIIB	T4, any N, M0 Any T, N3, M0
IV	Any T, any N, M1

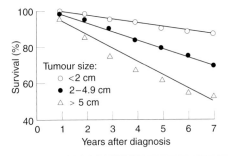

Fig. 22.6 Survival in relation to tumour size. (From: Dixon JM. ABC of Breast Diseases. London: BMJ Publishing Group 1995; p. 49, with permission.)

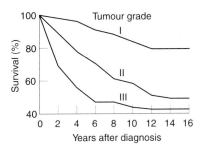

Fig. 22.7 Survival in relation to tumour grade. (From: Dixon JM. ABC of Breast Diseases. London: BMJ Publishing Group 1995; p. 26, with permission.)

An alternative is to use an integrated prognostic index such as the Nottingham Prognostic Index which combines tumour size, lymph node status and grade. The index is calculated by 0.2 × the tumour size (cm) + grade + lymph node stage (lymph node stage 1 if no nodes are involved, 2 if 1–3 nodes are involved and 3 if three or more nodes are involved). This separates patients into three prognostic groups: good, moderate and poor (Table 22.6).

Table 22.6 Nottingham Prognostic Index (NPI) and survival

Prognosis	NPI score	Survival (15 years)
Good	< 3.4	80%
Moderate	3.4–5.4	40%
Poor	> 5.4	15%

Other prognostic factors include the use of markers of proliferation. Patients with tumours that have a high rate of proliferation have an increased rate of local recurrence after mastectomy and a worse survival than patients whose tumours proliferate slowly. Several methods to measure proliferation have been reported, including the measurement of the fraction of the cells in the s-phase of the cell cycle, the use of monoclonal antibodies and the identification of proliferating cells by the use of tracers such as bromodeoxyuridine. Normal cells are diploid with regard to their DNA content. Many breast cancer cells have abnormal amounts of DNA and are aneuploid. Patients with aneuploid breast tumours have a worse prognosis than those with diploid tumours. The presence of oestrogen receptors in a breast cancer predicts response to hormonal manipulation and is also of some value in predicting early outcome after treatment but is of limited long-term prognostic value. The proto-oncogene, erbB2, or Her2 neu is overexpressed in 15–30% of invasive cancers and up to 80% of non-invasive cancers. Its product is homologous with the epidermal growth factor receptor. Patients with lymph node involvement whose tumours express erbB2 have a particularly poor prognosis. While erbB2 is of some value in delineating the prognosis of patients with lymph node-negative disease, its value in this group appears to be less. p53 is the product of a gene found on the short arm of chromosome 17. Its abnormal expression is the most common genetic lesion detected in breast cancers and loss of p53 is associated with a poor prognosis.

Although her overall prognosis is good, particularly in the short term, adjuvant therapy will reduce the risk of recurrence and will improve her overall survival. Adjuvant chemotherapy given for at least 3 months produces a highly significant 30% reduction in annual odds of recurrence in women aged under 50 and a 25% reduction in annual odds of death. Chemotherapy appears to be most effective in younger patients (Table 22.7). One-third or more of recurrences and one-quarter of all deaths in premenopausal women appear to be avoided or delayed by the use of adjuvant chemotherapy. Although this patient is at low risk of recurrence, options for adjuvant chemotherapy regimes are doxorubicin/cyclophosphamide (AC) or cyclophosphamide/methotrexate/5-fluorouracil (CMF) administered as an outpatient over a 3–6-month period.

Table 22.7 Reduction in recurrence and mortality in polychemotherapy trials

Age	Reduction in annual odds of recurrence (% ± SD)	Reduction in annual odds of death (% ± SD)
< 40	37 ± 7	27 ± 8
40–49	34 ± 5	27 ± 5
50–59	22 ± 4	14 ± 4
60–69	18 ± 4	8 ± 4
All ages	23 ± 8	15 ± 2

As her tumour is hormone receptor-positive, tamoxifen (20 mg a day for 5 years) should be considered. The benefit expected to accrue from tamoxifen in a premenopausal woman is an approximate 32% reduction in the annual odds of recurrence and death. If chemotherapy is to be given, the tamoxifen should be started after chemotherapy. Currently studies are assessing whether the addition of chemotherapy and hormonal therapy in premenopausal women reduces significantly the annual odds of recurrence and mortality to a greater degree than either alone. All decisions on treatment should be reached after a discussion with the patient covering likely benefits and side effects of different adjuvant therapies.

Table 22.8 Side effects from chemotherapy

• Low energy	Universal, fluctuates in relation to chemotherapy days
• Hair loss	Variable, inevitable with anthracyclines
• Nausea/vomiting	Mostly well controlled by 5 hydroxytryptamine ($5HT_3$) antagonists + steroid
• Mucositis	
• Gastritis	
• Weight gain	
• Increased appetite	Side effects of steroids
• Disturbed sleep	
• Neutropenia/sepsis	Approximately 5%. More common with anthracyclines
• Cardiomyopathy	Low but real risk (2–5%) with anthracyclines, especially Adriamycin. May be irreversible

The patient elects to receive systemic chemotherapy. How should the chemotherapy and breast irradiation be sequenced?

Although the difference in outcome would be small for the patient described, the optimal sequence of adjuvant therapy is for chemotherapy to be followed by radiation therapy. Several studies including a recent study from the Joint Center for Radiation Therapy in Boston showed an advantage for this sequence. The comparable rates for 5-year recurrence-free survival and survival without distant recurrence were 69% and 75% in those patients given chemotherapy first, compared to 62% and 64% for those who had radiotherapy first.

What side effects can she expect from the chemotherapy?

Complications and side effects of chemotherapy include alopecia, neutropenia, nausea and vomiting and early menopause (Table 22.8). Alopecia can be expected with high doses of cyclophosphamide and the most commonly used doses of doxorubicin (Adriamycin). Neutropenia is to be expected and regular blood checks should be performed. The nadir (lowest point) for most regimens is known. Delay of chemotherapy and dose reductions on subsequent cycles of therapy may be necessary if the white count falls below defined limits. Nausea and vomiting are among the more unpleasant side effects of chemotherapy. The percentage of patients experiencing nausea differs with the different combinations of chemotherapy and some regimens require few or no antiemetic measures. The arrival of the 3HT3 receptor antagonists has (at a cost) reduced the problem to manageable levels. It seems reasonable to reserve these agents for the more emetogenic regimens and for those whose nausea cannot be controlled by more routine measures such as regular metoclopramide, benzodiazapienes and dexamethasone. Young women (<40) are at greatest risk of nausea and vomiting following chemotherapy. The aim of treatment is to prevent them ever experiencing it so as to avoid the condition of anticipatory nausea and vomiting. A woman of age 42 is likely to have her menopausal age brought forward by receiving chemotherapy and most women in their late 40s receiving adjuvant chemotherapy will become menopausal by the end of treatment.

How often should patients attend for follow up after breast conservation?

Local recurrence in the treated breast occurs at a fixed rate of approximately 1% per year. Patients with carcinoma of one breast are also at an increased risk of cancer in the other breast and approximately 1% per year will develop this. All patients under follow up after breast conservation should have regular mammography with a baseline investigation 6–12 months after the initial surgery and mammograms of both breasts performed every year. Mammograms can be difficult to interpret after breast conservation because scarring from surgery can result in formation of a stellate opacity which can be difficult to differentiate from cancer recurrence. Ultrasound with the addition of colour Doppler is useful in making this differentiation. The most accurate of techniques in differentiating scar from recurrence is magnetic resonance imaging. By using a contrast agent the increased blood flow associated with tumour recurrence (demonstrated by gadolinium enhancement) is seen in contrast to the decreased flow (lack of enhancement) in areas of scar tissue. If recurrence is suspected, then a combination of further imaging, cytology and core biopsy may be necessary to confirm this.

Three years later, the patient is found on mammography to have two new areas of microcalcifications, one superior and the other at the site of the wide local excision. What is the differential diagnosis?

The differential diagnosis includes recurrent carcinoma, fat necrosis secondary to surgery and irradiation or calcifications due to benign breast disease, most commonly sclerosing adenosis. If the calcifications have a suspicious or indeterminate morphology, image-guided fine-needle aspiration cytology or core biopsy is indicated to obtain a definitive diagnosis.

A core biopsy of both areas demonstrates infiltrating carcinoma superior to the lumpectomy site and DCIS at the lumpectomy site. What are the options for local therapy?

Recurrent invasive carcinoma in a patient who has received breast irradiation is usually an indication for completion mastectomy. Breast 'recurrences' can be divided into true recurrences which occur at the tumour bed or new primaries which develop elsewhere in the breast. There is some very limited information to suggest that in patients who develop a new primary many years after treatment of the first cancer, adequate local control can be obtained by a further local excision. Standard practice for true recurrence or a second primary is, however, completion mastectomy. Patients should be checked for distant metastases as local recurrence is a risk factor for distant relapse. In one study, local relapse was associated with a 3.4 times greater risk of distant relapse. Time to relapse is also important and the later the local recurrence occurs, the better the outlook (Table 22.9).

Table 22.9 Significance of local recurrence

Time to relapse	Number of patients	Number with distant metastases
<5 years	191	109
>5 years	49	9

She wishes to be considered for breast reconstruction after the mastectomy. What are the options?

Reconstruction of an irradiated breast should be performed using autologous tissue rather than using expanders/implants since high

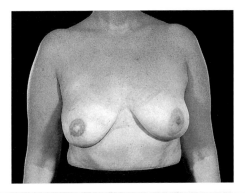

Fig. 22.8 Patient who has had a TRAM flap reconstruction.

rates of complications are reported when implants or expanders are used in this situation. The reconstructive options are either a TRAM flap, pedicled or free (Figure 22.8), or a latissimus dorsi myocutaneous flap and implant (Figure 22.9). The former has the benefit of the reconstruction consisting entirely of autologous tissue but the disadvantage is that it involves considerably more dissection, and potentially more risks and complications.

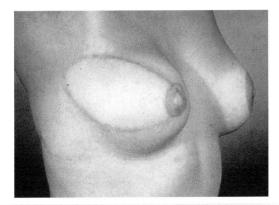

Fig. 22.9 Patient who has had a latissimus dorsi reconstruction. There is an implant under the muscle and this patient had a nipple reconstruction.

The gold standard breast reconstruction is the TRAM flap. When first introduced, the TRAM flap was used as a pedicled flap based on the superior epigastric artery. However, this is not the dominant blood supply of the skin island that is used, which comes from the infra-umbilical area. The greater blood supply to this area is from the inferior epigastric artery (Figure 22.10) and is the vessel used when the flap is transferred by microvascular means (free TRAM flap). More

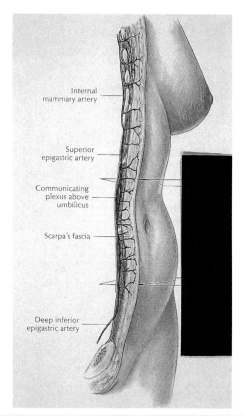

Fig. 22.10 Blood supply from inferior epigastric artery for a TRAM flap.
(From: Bostwick J. Plastic and Reconstructive Breast Surgery. Vol. II.
Quality Medical Publishing, Inc., St Louis, 1990. p. 786.)

recently, a technique has been described in which the skin/fat of the
flap is dissected out on its vascular pedicle without including part of
the rectus muscle. This avoids the potential complication of abdominal
wall weakness/hernae which has been reported following free and
pedicled TRAM flaps and avoids the need for synthetic replacement of
the rectus sheath. As with all free tissue transfers, failure to
revascularize the flap is a potential complication which occurs in up to
5% of patients. When the TRAM flap is pedicled, major necrosis occurs
in up to 10%. Patient selection is of great importance when trying to
reduce necrosis rates to a minimum. Smokers, patients who have had
previous radiotherapy, those with diabetes mellitus and obese patients
are at particular risk of flap loss from a single pedicled TRAM flap. Such
patients should be considered for either a bipedicled flap raised on
both superior epigastric vessels or a free flap. Any previous surgical
operation which has divided the superior epigastric artery is an

absolute contraindication for the pedicled technique. TRAM flaps are major operations and, although they can produce a satisfactory cosmetic result, they do leave major scarring, particularly on the abdomen (Figure 22.8).

The latissimus dorsi myocutaneous flap (LD flap) is, from a vascular point of view, the most reliable of the pedicled flaps. Major skin necrosis affects less than 1% of patients. The problem with the LD flap is that in almost every patient it is necessary to use an implant. It also results in a scar on the back which, unless it is carefully situated, can be difficult to hide when wearing low-backed clothes (Figure 22.11). When using an implant there are the problems of implant type, possible infection and capsular contracture. Overall, it does, however, produce satisfactory results in most patients.

There is no evidence that immediate reconstruction increases the rate of local or systemic relapse and it reduces the psychological trauma of change in body image experienced after mastectomy. Immediate breast reconstruction appears to be associated with substantially better cosmetic and psychological outcomes than delayed reconstruction and should be more widely available than it is at present.

It is important to ascertain the woman's expectations from a reconstruction. These must be realistic. It is not possible to replace that which has been lost with an exact copy. Frequently more than one operation is required. It may be necessary to carry out a contralateral breast reduction or to correct the ptosis of the opposite breast (mastopexy). These should be mentioned early in discussions about the reconstruction process.

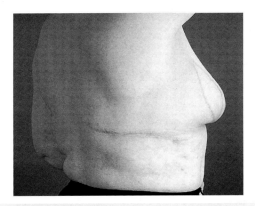

Fig. 22.11 Back scar from latissimus dorsi flap.

Once an adequate breast mound has been achieved, some women will want to consider nipple reconstruction or, more correctly, nipple areolar complex reconstruction (Figure 22.9). The areola is usually made using a full thickness skin graft from an area of relatively dark skin, e.g. upper inner thigh or by sharing the remaining contralateral areola. Alternatively it can be recreated by tattooing. The nipple prominence can be made from local skin or by nipple sharing. The latter gives a better colour match but may not be possible in all women. Prosthetic nipples are available for those who do not wish further surgery.

The patient undergoes completion mastectomy with TRAM flap reconstruction. The mastectomy specimen demonstrates extensive DCIS in all quadrants, and a 0.6 cm grade 1 infiltrating ductal carcinoma. Is additional adjuvant therapy warranted?

The residual focus of invasive cancer (0.6 cm) was detected in the same quadrant of the breast as the original tumour. It could be reasonably argued that the invasive disease now present represents either residual disease from the original tumour or a new primary tumour. In either case, the disease has been adequately treated with a mastectomy and there is no further advantage to be gained by additional adjuvant therapy. No data on giving chemotherapy in this situation are available. There is, however, a problem in patients who have extensive recurrent disease and, in this situation, following a discussion with the patient, further chemotherapy may be deemed appropriate.

A patient who presents with increasing distortion and superficial ulceration at the site of a wide excision and post-operative radiotherapy

J M Dixon

A woman presents 15 years after receiving a wide local excision and radiotherapy with an iridium wire boost, complaining of increasing distortion of the latter aspect of her breast and some superficial ulceration (Figure 23.1). What is the likely cause and how should it be treated?

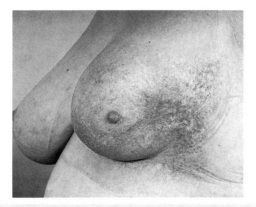

Fig. 23.1 Area of distortion of the latter aspect of left breast and some superficial ulceration due to radiation damage.

The two possible causes are radiotherapy damage to the tissues or recurrent cancer. The photograph is more characteristic of radiation damage. Details of the dose of radiotherapy should be obtained. This patient had a total dose of 45 Gy to the whole breast with a 30 Gy local boost giving a total dose of 75 Gy to the tumour bed. This is a large dose and would explain the local effects.

The area causes her increasing pain, and the ulceration has been present for some time and shows no signs of healing. What are the surgical options for this patient?

This area of damaged tissue needs to be excised. This can be performed either as a total mastectomy or as a wide excision of the localized area which received the 75 Gy of radiotherapy with the defect in the breast being closed by a myocutaneous flap (Figure 23.2). Figure 23.2 demonstrates the final result in this patient following removal of the damaged tissue and a latissimus dorsi myocutaneous flap reconstruction. The cosmetic result has improved as has the nipple position and this totally relieved the pain.

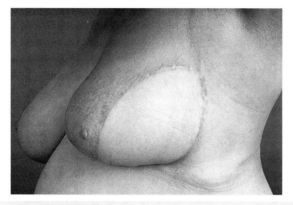

Fig. 23.2 Area of damaged tissue excised and the defect in the breast closed by a latissimus dorsi flap.

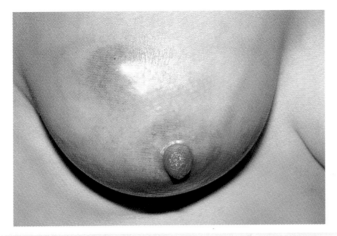

Figure 10.2 Lactating breast abscess.

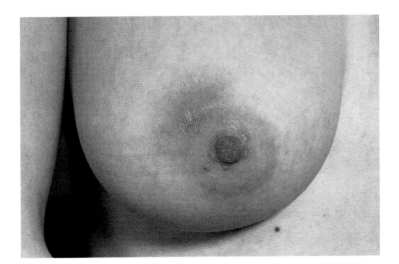

Figure 11.1 Periareolar inflammation secondary to periductal mastitis.

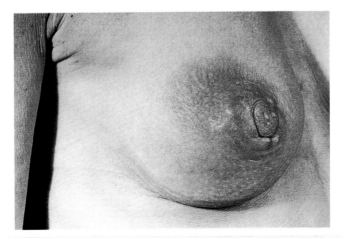

Figure 11.2 Periareolar abscess secondary to periductal mastitis.

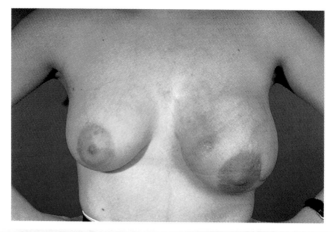

Figure 16.1 Patient with a recurrent malignant phyllodes tumour in the left breast.

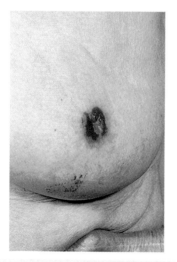

Figure 18.1 Paget's disease of the nipple.

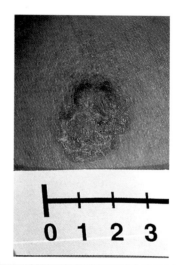

Figure 18.2 Eczema of the nipple.

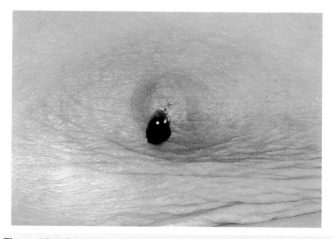

Figure 18.4 Bloodstained nipple discharge.

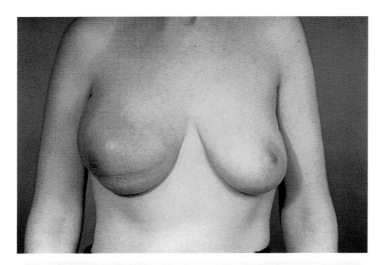

Figure 28.1 Inflammatory cancer affecting the right breast.

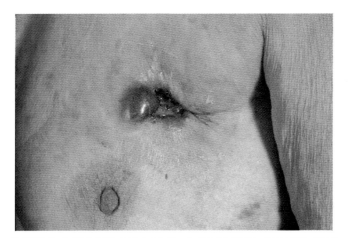

Figure 29.1 Ulcerated locally advanced breast cancer.

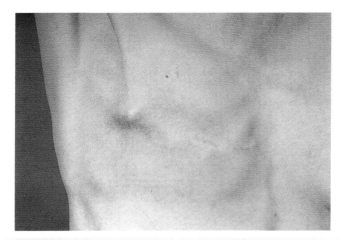

Figure 32.1 Single spot recurrence after mastectomy.

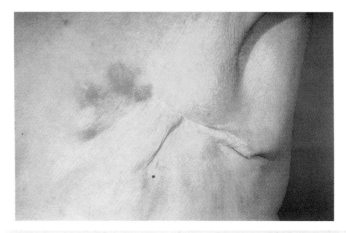

Figure 32.2 Multiple spot recurrence after mastectomy.

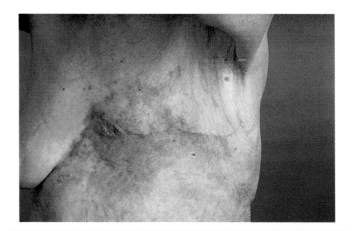

Figure 32.3 Field recurrence after mastectomy.

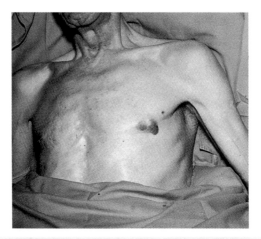

Figure 33.1 A male with breast cancer.

A 45-year-old premenopausal woman who presents with a 3.2 cm mass in the right breast with skin dimpling

W Gradishar and M Morrow

A 45-year-old premenopausal women presents with a 3-week history of a right breast lump. On examination she has a 3.2 cm mass in the right breast with skin dimpling and firm mobile nodes in the axilla. What investigations would you perform to establish the diagnosis?

A mammogram with magnification of the tumour site should be obtained and a needle biopsy technique should be used to establish the diagnosis of carcinoma. Patients with contraindications to breast-conserving therapy can be identified with a careful history, clinical examination and magnification mammography in 95% of cases, eliminating inappropriate attempts to perform lumpectomy in patients who require mastectomy. The criteria for breast conservation are listed in Table 22.1. Patients with operable breast cancer who are best treated by mastectomy are those who prefer mastectomy, those who would achieve a poor cosmetic result from breast conservation, patients with multiple cancers, and patients with multiple risk factors for local recurrence.

If cancer is confirmed, are there any other investigations you would undertake?

A chest X-ray should be performed and blood should be removed for a full blood count, liver functions tests and serum calcium. The utility of bone scanning in this circumstance is controversial and in the absence of symptoms a bone scan would not be indicated. Bone scans in asymptomatic patients with stage 1 and 2 breast cancer identify metastatic disease in fewer than 5% of cases. False-positive studies are common and areas of abnormality on a scan must be investigated with plain radiographs. Other imaging studies such as liver scans or CT scans of the abdomen or brain are even less likely to identify disease in asymptomatic patients and should not be performed.

Assuming all the investigations are normal, how would you stage this patient's breast cancer?

She has a clinical T_2, N_1-stage IIb carcinoma. This determination is based on the fact that the tumour size is between 2 and 5 cm and there is clinically suspicious lymphadenopathy. The presence of skin dimpling is related to the location of the tumour within the breast and is not a prognostic factor which impacts upon stage. The TNM staging system for breast cancer is shown in Table 22.5a.

If the cancer is confirmed and there is no obvious evidence of metastases, what are the options for treatment for this patient?

Whether or not this patient is an appropriate candidate for breast-conserving therapy is dependent on the size of the tumour relative to the size of the breast. In the patient with a very small breast, cosmesis is unlikely to be satisfactory after excision of 3.2 cm tumour. The use of preoperative chemotherapy increases rates of breast conserving therapy in patients with larger tumours but this should not be regarded as standard therapy at the present time.

The observed kinetic acceleration of micrometastatic disease following non-curative surgical excision in animal studies is strong biological evidence to support primary chemotherapy. Primary chemotherapy has been reported in one study to reduce the frequency of mastectomy in women with tumours initially considered too large for breast-conserving therapy, although in the randomized trial conducted by the NSABP of preoperative versus post-operative chemotherapy, breast-conservation rates were increased by only 8% in the primary chemotherapy group. From studies of various drug combinations, it appears that the incidence of pathological complete remission remains 10% or less. Based on results from Milan, it appears that the degree of tumour response is a marker of treatment outcome, at least for the first 5 years. However, randomized trials of primary chemotherapy versus post-operative treatment have so far failed to show a survival benefit for the primary systemic therapy approach.

Table 24.1 Advantages of primary systemic therapy

	Primary systemic therapy	Post-operative therapy
Advantages	Assess antitumour activity	Known benefits following years of follow up in thousands of patients
	Downstage & achieve conservation	Axillary node status for prognosis
Disadvantages*	No information on axillary nodes	Benefit for individual patient unknown

*Assumes core or wedge biopsy performed to assess primary tumour pathology and ER status.

A high complete remission rate might be expected by combining doxorubicin and paclitaxel but there are few published studies on this combination. Despite the logical and scientific rationale and the theoretical advantages of primary systemic therapy (Table 24.1), available data do not as yet provide sufficient evidence to indicate a clear superiority of primary chemotherapy over adjuvant chemotherapy. The other question to answer through prospective randomized trials is not whether the shift from adjuvant to neo-adjuvant chemotherapy will result in a superior outcome, but rather how to integrate primary and adjuvant drug regimens properly to maximize tumour cell kill.

The presence of skin dimpling and palpable adenopathy are not contraindications to breast-conserving therapy unless the nodes are fixed. When skin dimpling is due to a very superficially located tumour, excision of the dimpled skin may be necessary to ensure a negative margin. Positive axillary nodes are an indicator of a high risk of systemic relapse but they are not associated with an increased risk of breast recurrence following breast conservation.

If the patient's breasts are small relative to the size of the tumour or mammograms show disease elsewhere, the patient may be a candidate for a modified radical mastectomy alone, with or without immediate reconstruction. If reconstruction is chosen, the use of autologous tissue reconstruction is preferred because, if the patient has more than four positive nodes in the axilla then she would be at increased risk of chest wall recurrence and would be a candidate for chest wall irradiation to reduce the risk of locoregional relapse. Factors which increase the rates of chest wall relapse after mastectomy are listed in Table 24.2. Patients who have more than four axillary lymph nodes

Table 24.2 Indications for radiotherapy after mastectomy

- More than four axillary nodes positive
- Direct involvement of the fascia or muscle underlying the breast
- Lymphatic/vascular invasion
- Grade 3 tumour
- Pathological tumour size > 4 cm

positive or those with direct involvement of the fascia or muscle, or patients with two of the other three factors are candidates for radiotherapy.

Because tumour size is not a risk factor for local recurrence, the only reason for treating large tumours by mastectomy is because, once they have been excised, the cosmetic result is unsatisfactory. It is now possible to replace quite large volumes of tissue using a latissimus dorsi muscle flap and overlying fat. This latissimus dorsi mini-flap can be raised without a skin incision over the back and produces satisfactory cosmetic results. To be oncologically safe it is best performed in two procedures. The first operation is a wide local excision and, providing the lesion has been satisfactorily removed histologically, then thereafter an axillary node dissection combined with a latissimus dorsi mini-flap can be performed a few days later. This ensures that the defect in the breast does not have time to contract. The final cosmetic result is shown in Figures 24.1a and b.

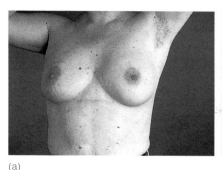
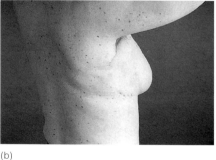

(a)   (b)

Fig. 24.1 Patient who has had a very wide excision of a 6 cm carcinoma with the defect in the breast filled with a latissimus dorsi mini-flap. Views from front (a) and back (b).

You elect to treat her by breast conservation and the pathology demonstrates a 2.8 cm grade III cancer which appears completely excised. Four out of 21 axillary lymph nodes are involved and the tumour is oestrogen receptor-negative. What are the options for adjuvant treatment in this patient?

This premenopausal patient has a pathologic stage IIb invasive breast cancer (see Table 22.5b). Adjuvant therapy must include both breast irradiation combined with systemic chemotherapy. For this patient, the 5-year risk of recurrence and mortality is approximately 50%. She is therefore considered at high risk (Table 24.3). A summary of prescription of adjuvant therapy for different risk groups is presented in Table 24.4. Since the risk of systemic disease is significantly greater for patients with multiple involved axillary lymph nodes, systemic adjuvant chemotherapy should precede the administration of radiotherapy. Adjuvant chemotherapy programmes that would be considered appropriate for this patient include AC, CMF, or AC followed by CMF. Bonadonna compared in a prospective randomized study the effectiveness of four courses of doxorubicin following by eight courses of CMF with two courses of CMF alternating with one course of doxorubicin for a total of 12 courses. All drug courses were recycled every 3 weeks and the median duration of follow up at the time of analysis was 9 years. A total of 405 women were entered into the study, 403 of whom met the protocol criteria. Patient characteristics were well balanced between the two treatment groups with the exception of

Table 24.3 Risk definitions

	Grade	Size	Nodal status
Very low risk	1	<2 cm	Node −ve
Low risk	1	>2 cm	Node −ve
	2	<2 cm	Node −ve
Moderate risk	1	Any	Node +ve
	2	>2 cm	Node −ve
	3	<5 cm	Node −ve
High risk	2	Any	Node +ve
	3	>5 cm	Node −ve
	3	Any	1–3 nodes +ve
Very high risk	3	Any	>4 nodes +ve

Table 24.4 Summary of prescription of adjuvant therapy for different risk groups

Risk group	Adjuvant therapy advised
Premenopausal	
Very low risk	Nil or trial of tamoxifen
Low risk ER + ve	Tamoxifen ± ovarian suppression
Low risk ER − ve	CMF or AC chemotherapy
Moderate risk ER + ve	CMF or AC + tamoxifen ± ovarian ablation
Moderate risk ER − ve	CMF or anthracycline
High/very high risk	Anthracycline or high-dose trial
Post-menopausal	
Very low risk	Nil or tamoxifen trial
Low risk ER + ve	Tamoxifen
Moderate risk	Tamoxifen ± CMF
Moderate risk ER − ve	CMF ± tamoxifen
High/very high risk (younger)	Anthracycline or high-dose trial
High/very high risk (older 60 +)	CMF or anthracycline

ER, oestrogen receptor; CMF, cytophosphamide/methotrexate/5-fluorouracil; AC, aoxorubicin/cyclophosphamide.

the extent of nodal involvement: 38% had more than ten positive nodes in the alternating regime compared to 29% in the sequential regimen, and this difference was not statistically significant. The results of this study demonstrated a significantly superior survival for patients who received the sequential regimen, four cycles of AC followed by eight cycles of CMF compared to those given alternating chemotherapy. The relapse-free survival was 42% versus 28% ($p = 0.002$) and the total survival was 58% versus 44% ($p = 0.002$, respectively). The benefit of the sequential regimen was evident in all patient subsets. Treatment was fairly well tolerated but four cases of congestive cardiac failure were documented and these were fatal in two patients. They concluded that, in women with extensive nodal involvement, sequential chemotherapy with doxorubicin followed by CMF yielded superior results compared with alternating administration of the same regimens. They also compared their results with a retrospective series of patients treated with the classical CMF regimen and, although not a direct comparison, sequential therapy appeared to produce superior results to classical CMF.

New drugs with significant activity in the metastatic disease setting, such as taxanes (paclitaxel, docetaxel), are currently being incorporated into adjuvant chemotherapy programmes but their use at present should be limited to clinical trials. Another investigational treatment strategy that could be considered in this relatively high-risk patient is the use of dose-escalation chemotherapy followed by peripheral blood stem cell support. Although no definitive data yet exist clarifying the role of high-dose chemotherapy in the treatment of breast cancer, a few reports have suggested a better outcome for high-risk patients (>10 involved axillary lymph nodes) treated with high-dose chemotherapy compared to standard-dose chemotherapy. High-dose chemotherapy in this situation, however, should only be given as part of ongoing clinical trials. Exact details of the level of her oestrogen receptor would need to be obtained. If her tumour was oestrogen-receptor zero, then tamoxifen therapy would not be recommended. If on the other hand the tumour had a small percentage of cells staining, and the receptor was low but not zero, then tamoxifen is appropriate. Patients can be classified into different risk groups based on node status and other histological factors (Table 24.3). Although not widely used, for oestrogen receptor-positive patients oophorectomy is at least as effective as chemotherapy and in a Scottish study which compared CMF chemotherapy with oophorectomy, patients who were oestrogen receptor-positive had a better relapse-free survival with oophorectomy, whereas patients who were oestrogen receptor-negative had a better relapse-free survival with chemotherapy (Figure 24.2).

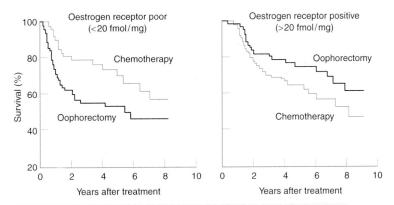

Fig. 24.2 Comparison of CMF chemotherapy with oophorectomy based on ER status. (From: Dixon JM. ABC of Breast Diseases. London: BMJ Publishing Group 1995; p. 56, with permission.)

She receives six courses of adjuvant CMF chemotherapy but returns 18 months later with weight loss, and right upper quadrant tenderness. What is the likely diagnosis and how would you establish this?

The new symptoms of abdominal pain and weight loss raise the concern that metastatic liver disease has developed. Although liver function tests should be ordered, imaging of the right upper quadrant by ultrasonography or computed tomography is indicated. In addition, restaging of other sites should be performed at this time including chest X-ray and bone scan. Any other abnormalities detected on history and clinical examination should also be evaluated at this time. Although it is a common dictum that new metastatic disease should be confirmed by biopsy, the radiological appearance of the liver may leave little doubt that metastatic disease is present. All single lesions should be confirmed by needle-aspiration cytology or core biopsy. Likewise, if there is doubt on radiological investigations, a histological or cytological diagnosis should be performed before treatment is undertaken. Alternatively, if there is a more accessible lesion on clinical examination, such as an enlarged lymph node, then fine-needle aspiration cytology or core biopsy should be performed from this site, as biopsying locoregional disease is associated with potentially less morbidity.

Having established she has liver metastases, what options are available for treatment and what is the likely response?

Unfortunately, this patient now has metastatic cancer and is unlikely to be cured by any form of therapy, although systemic chemotherapy has a good chance of slowing the tempo of the disease and improving symptoms related to the disease. The median survival for patients presenting with metastatic disease is less than 2 years, although patients with disease predominantly in soft tissues or bone can live considerably longer (Figure 24.3). In a patient who has already received treatment with CMF in the adjuvant setting, a treatment regimen containing doxorubicin, a taxane or both would be a reasonable choice. There is evidence that the duration of response is longer with combination chemotherapy than with single agents but duration of response of single agents given sequentially is clinically equivalent. In addition, single-agent doxorubicin, paclitaxel or docetaxel, using the maximum tolerated dose, may provide the same

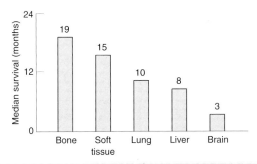

Fig. 24.3 Median time of survival associated with site of metastasis in patients with breast cancer. (From: Dixon JM. ABC of Breast Diseases. London: BMJ Publishing Group 1995; p. 45, with permission.)

range of response rates in metastatic breast cancer to that obtained with combination chemotherapy regimens. The choice of a combination regimen or a single agent is based on the patient's previous exposure to chemotherapy and response to chemotherapy. The commonly recommended strategy for the use of chemotherapy in a patient with metastatic disease who has not yet been previously treated is to use one of the various CMF regimens or, alternatively, a doxorubicin-based regimen as first-line treatment. Upon progression with CMF, single-agent therapy with doxorubicin at a dose of $60–75 \ mg/m^2$ every 3 weeks or epirubicin at a equivalent dose, i.e. $60 \ mg/m^2$ would be reasonable choices. Third-line chemotherapy options include a taxane, such as paclitaxel, $175 \ mg/m^2$ in a 3-hour i.v. infusion every 3 weeks or docetaxel $100 \ mg/m^2$, given as a 1-hour infusion every 3 weeks. The chance of a response to any further chemotherapy after these regimens have been utilized is very small, although sometimes the same drug which worked previously can be effective on re-introduction, especially if a long period of time has passed or a different schedule is employed. A typical example is the use of 5-fluorouracil (5-FU) given as a continuous infusion in patients who have previously received this drug as part of the cyclophosphamide, adriamycin and 5-fluorouracil (CAF-) or CMF-type combination, or a long infusion of paclitaxel in patients progressing on short paclitaxel courses.

The optimal duration of chemotherapy in responding patients has yet to be defined. Maintenance chemotherapy beyond achievement of a complete or partial remission provides little or no survival benefit. When maximal tumour response is achieved, many clinicians give one additional cycle to confirm stabilization and maximal response, and then discontinue chemotherapy. When the tumour then progresses at a later stage, chemotherapy is then reinstituted. Randomized prospective trials have shown that the survival of patients treated according to this strategy is equivalent to that of patients receiving continuous chemotherapy and the intermittent strategy produces less toxicity. A critical issue is to balance symptoms from the cancer, after maximal remission is achieved, and the toxicity of chemotherapy. If the patient still has significant symptoms after partial response, chemotherapy should be continued. If symptoms are minimal or absent and toxicity is significant, chemotherapy can be discontinued. The expected tumour response rate to doxorubicin or a taxane in a patient with liver metastases who has been previously treated with CMF is in the range of 30–40%.

The potential clinical benefits of high-dose chemotherapy with haemopoietic support in the treatment of metastatic breast cancer include a high complete remission rate and prolonged disease-free survival in approximately one in five women. On the other hand, high-dose chemotherapy is very toxic, is associated with a small mortality rate and selection of patients included in trials may well have had an influence on results. These observations, coupled with the fact that most of the data available have been generated from uncontrolled, single-institution pilot studies indicates that high-dose chemotherapy should be used only as part of ongoing prospective trials. Results of two small randomized trials comparing conventional chemotherapy with high-dose chemotherapy and metastatic breast cancer have so far been reported. The first trial compared tandem high-dose chemotherapy with conventional chemotherapy and showed an increased complete response rate, disease-free and overall survival in women randomized to the high-dose arm. Criticisms of this trial include the inclusion of only small numbers of patients, the use of suboptimal chemotherapy in the conventional dose arm and a greater use of tamoxifen in women treated in the high-dose arm. In another recent randomized trial, high-dose treatment gave better results when used at the time of relapse following a complete remission after conventional dose chemotherapy than when used immediately on achieving complete remission. The areas of current research in high-dose chemotherapy include the definition of optimal regimens, the integration of new agents, the timing of high-dose chemotherapy and the worth of tandem multiple cycles of high-dose chemotherapy.

Biological therapies have been a focus of intense research in breast cancer. Promising preclinical studies have led to clinical trials exploring the use of monoclonal antibodies directed against growth factor receptors, anticarcinogenic agents and other strategies such as vaccines. Administration of antibodies to the putative growth factor erbB2–HER 2/neu in patients with metastatic breast cancer overexpressing the *her 2/neu* oncogene can cause prolonged remission. Recently reported clinical trials indicate that the use of these antibodies in patients with advanced breast cancer produces a major response in approximately 12% of patients. Another growth factor receptor that can be exploited as a specific target in cancer therapy is the epidermal growth factor receptor. These biological approaches may have a role in combination with chemotherapy regimens and are currently being tested in randomized clinical trials.

25 A 58-year-old woman who presents with a lump in her breast of 6-months' duration

J M Dixon and R C F Leonard

Mrs M is a 58-year-old who has been aware of a lump in her breast for 6 months. She is post-menopausal and currently not on hormone replacement therapy. On examination there is an obvious mass visible in her left breast. There is some skin tethering and mobile palpable nodes in the left axilla which are not obviously malignant. When you see her at the clinic, what should you tell her?

Clinical examination alone does not have a 100% accuracy even in a patient of 65. A number of conditions can produce skin dimpling, including previous surgery, fat necrosis and sclerosing lesions. Having said that, this constellation of signs is unlikely to be due to anything but a breast cancer. You should tell her that you are very suspicious that this lump is not straightforward. Having given her time to ask exactly what this means, you then either answer any questions she poses or state that you think the lump is likely to be a growth or a tumour. Some clinicians omit the comment about the lump not being straightforward and move straight to this statement. The patient may ask what type of tumour it is, and it would then be appropriate to tell her that you think it is likely to be a cancer but that you need definite proof.

Subsequent investigations confirm a cancer measuring 4.5 cm in maximum diameter as measured by callipers. Mammograms demonstrate a stellate mass lesion measuring 3.8 cm in maximum dimension. A core biopsy taken in the clinic establishes that this is a grade II cancer which is strongly oestrogen receptor-positive with a histoscore of 270. (This means it is a tumour which is highly oestrogen receptor-positive.) A score of 80 is roughly equivalent to

20 fmol/mg cytosol protein. What are the options for treatment of this patient?

The surgical options depend on the size of her breast. Excising a 4.5 cm from most women's breasts would leave an unacceptable cosmetic result. If, however, the patient has a large breast, it may be possible to widely excise such a cancer and leave a reasonable result. There are technical problems giving post-operative radiotherapy to large breasts and any decision to proceed with breast conservation should be taken only after consultation with a radiation oncologist. There are techniques available whereby large, unifocal cancers can be excised and the resultant defect in the breast replaced by a latissimus dorsi mini-flap, but these remain experimental. The standard option in this patient would be a mastectomy combined with an axillary clearance. Subsequent systemic therapy would then be based on the histology of the primary tumour and the histological status of the axillary lymph nodes.

An alternative option in this patient would be to treat her with a 3-month course of primary systemic therapy in the hope of reducing her tumour size and making breast conservation possible. This is not standard treatment, however, and primary systemic therapy should be restricted to units undertaking clinical trials. The standard practice in most units using systemic therapy for large operable breast cancers has been to treat patients irrespective of their oestrogen receptor status with neo-adjuvant chemotherapy. It has been demonstrated however, that, in a patient who has a high oestrogen-receptor content, there is a high probability (>90%) that the tumour will respond to primary hormonal treatment such as tamoxifen. The average reduction in volume over 3 months is over 50% and can permit wide excision in approximately 75% of such patients without the associated side effects of chemotherapy (Figure 25.1). Recent studies using aromatase inhibitors as primary treatment in post-menopausal women with large, operable, oestrogen-receptor breast cancers have produced similar promising results (Figure 25.2) and further investigation of the use of these agents in this setting are proceeding. During primary systemic therapy, patients should be assessed at monthly intervals by both clinical examination and ultrasound (Figure 25.3) and, at the end of the treatment period (usually 3 months), they should have repeat mammography (Figure 25.4). Although treatment can be continued to maximum response, most units treat patients for a fixed time interval,

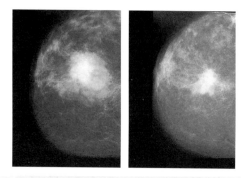

Fig. 25.1 Mammograms before (left) and after tamoxifen treatment (right).

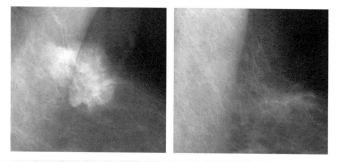

Fig. 25.2 Mammograms before (left) and after letrozole treatment (right).

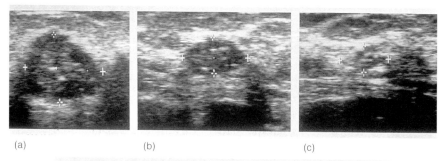

(a) (b) (c)

Fig. 25.3 Ultrasound (a) before, (b) one month after and (c) three months after primary systemic therapy.

the aim being to obtain sufficient reduction in tumour volume to allow less surgery and to determine that the tumour is sensitive to that particular therapy so the same treatment can be continued after surgery. There is no published evidence that primary systemic therapy is associated with an improvement in survival when compared with standard treatment.

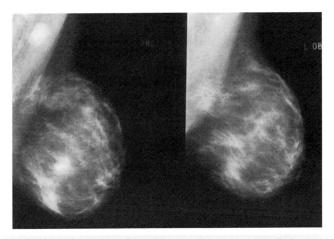

Fig. 25.4 Mammograms before (left) and after primary systemic therapy (right), showing disappearance of both the breast mass and axillary node.

All patients, irrespective of age, who have operable breast cancer and are fit for surgery should be treated within standard protocols. The use of tamoxifen alone for long periods in elderly patients is not appropriate other than in the small group of women where surgery is not an option. In reality, the number of patients who are unfit for surgery is very small as wide local excision, axillary clearance and mastectomy can be performed under local or regional anaesthesia.

Mastectomy is performed and demonstrates a 3.5 cm grade II breast cancer without lymphatic/vascular invasion and without axillary node involvement. What adjuvant therapy would you give her?

She would not be a candidate for post-operative chest-wall radiotherapy as she is not deemed at increased risk of local recurrence (see Table 24.2). Adjuvant systemic therapy in a post-menopausal node-negative patient is prescribed on the basis of calculated risk of recurrence (see Table 24.3). This patient falls into the moderate risk category, and options for adjuvant therapy are, therefore, tamoxifen alone or tamoxifen combined with chemotherapy (see Table 24.4). The benefits in terms of odds of reduction of risk of recurrence and absolute survival benefits for post-menopausal women given tamoxifen subdivided by oestrogen receptor and length of time on tamoxifen are shown in Table 25.1. The importance of giving 5 years of tamoxifen and the role of ER are clear from these data. The benefits of tamoxifen related to age are shown in Table 25.4. The benefits of giving

Table 25.1 Odds reduction of risk of recurrence and absolute survival benefits for post-menopausal patients given tamoxifen subdivided by oestrogen receptor

	Recurrence [% (SD)]	Death [% (SD)]
Tamoxifen 1 year		
ER poor (< 10 fmol/mg)	6 (8)	6 (8)
ER unknown	20 (4)	10 (4)
ER-positive	21 (5)	14 (5)
Tamoxifen 2 years		
ER poor	13 (5)	7 (5)
ER unknown	28 (4)	15 (4)
ER-positive	28 (3)	18 (4)
Tamoxifen 5 years		
ER poor	6 (11)	−3 (11)
ER unknown	37 (8)	21 (9)
ER-positive	50 (4)	28 (5)

ER, oestrogen receptor.
Adapted from Early Breast Cancer Trialists' Collaborative Group. Tamoxifen for early breast cancer: an overview of the randomised trials. Lancet 1998; 351: 1451–1467 © by The Lancet Ltd.

chemotherapy or tamoxifen alone or the two combined are listed in Table 25.2. Gains from chemotherapy in terms of odds reduction in recurrence or death are significant, although less likely than those from 5 years of tamoxifen. More data on the effectiveness of combining chemotherapy and tamoxifen are presented in Table 25.3. The decision whether to add chemotherapy to 5 years of tamoxifen in this patient should be taken after discussion with the patient of the likely benefits of this treatment.

Table 25.2 Benefits of chemotherapy or tamoxifen or a combination of chemotherapy and tamoxifen

Allocated treatment	Proportion reduction in annual mortality [% (SD)]	Absolute reduction in 10-year mortality per 100 women treated [% (SD)]
Age ⩾50 years		
(i) Polychemotherapy alone (e.g. ⩾6 months CMF)	12 (4)	5 (2)
(ii) Tamoxifen alone (for a median of 2 years)	20 (2)	8 (1)
(iii) Polychemotherapy + tamoxifen	30 (5)	12 (2)

Table 25.3 Gains from chemotherapy in terms of odds reduction in post-menopausal patients

Type of study	Reduction (SD) in annual odds	
	Recurrence	Death
Chemotherapy and tamoxifen versus tamoxifen	26% (5)	10% (7)
Chemotherapy and tamoxifen versus chemotherapy	28% (3)	20% (4)

Adapted from Early Breast Cancer Trialists' Collaborative Group. Systemic treatment of early breast cancer by hormonal, cytotoxic, or immune therapy. Lancet 1992; 339: 1, 71 © by The Lancet Ltd.

Table 25.4 Proportional risk reductions subdivided into age groups after exclusion of patients with oestrogen receptor-poor disease

Tamoxifen 5 years	Proportional reduction in annual odds of recurrence [% (SD)]	Proportional reduction in annual odds of death [% (SD)]
Age <50 92% ER+	45 (8)	32 (10)
Age 50–59 93% ER+	37 (6)	11 (8)
Age 60–69 95% ER+	54 (5)	33 (6)
Age 70+ 94% ER+	54 (13)	34 (13)
Overall 94% ER+	47 (3)	26 (4)

What complications can occur after mastectomy?

Common complications after mastectomy include the formation of a seroma, infection or flap necrosis. Collection of fluid under mastectomy flaps after suction drains have been removed (seromas) occur in between a third and half of all patients. Seromas are more common after modified radical mastectomy where the axillary nodes are removed than after mastectomy alone. Seromas can be aspirated if troublesome. Infection after mastectomy is uncommon and, when it occurs, it is usually secondary to flap necrosis. Rarely, areas of necrotic skin need to be excised and skin grafts applied. Most patients treated by mastectomy are suitable for some form of breast reconstruction which should ideally be performed at the same time as the initial mastectomy.

It the patient had wished to consider immediate breast reconstruction. What would have been her options?

As well as the options for myocutaneous flaps which were discussed previously (TRAM, see earlier), the use of tissue expansion as a reconstructive option should be considered. Tissue expansion involves the insertion of an expander in a submuscular pocket at the time of mastectomy. After the wound has healed, the device is inflated using saline, usually at weekly intervals. When the desired volume is achieved, the tissues are allowed to stabilize for some months. Most surgeons inflate with a greater volume of saline than the estimated final prosthesis volume to recreate a degree of breast ptosis when the definitive implant is inserted (Figure 25.5). It is current practice to use textured silicone gel-filled implants, although some (particularly in the USA) favour saline-filled prostheses. The texturing of the surface of the implant reduces the incidence of capsular contraction. This greatly enhances the aesthetic result. Despite the use of overexpansion, it is extremely difficult to create breast ptosis using this technique. A second operation is required when the expander is removed and a definitive prosthesis inserted. The time interval between the two can be as much as 6 months (Figure 25.6). In certain circumstances, it is appropriate to use an expander/prosthesis (Becker), thereby avoiding a second operation requiring a general anaesthetic. The expander

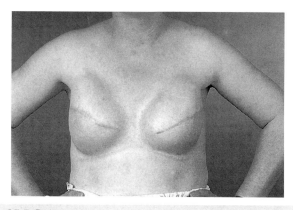

Fig. 25.5 Patient with overinflated bilateral tissue expanders *in situ.*

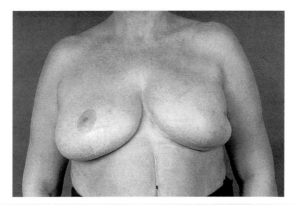

Fig. 25.6 Cosmetic result following replacement of a tissue expander with a permanent prosthesis. This patient has also had a right-sided reduction mammoplasty.

prosthesis consists of two envelopes, an outer layer of silicone and an inner envelope, which is filled through a remote filler port with saline. It is overexpanded and left for 2–3 months; thereafter the volume is adjusted by removing saline through the injection port until symmetry is obtained. Subsequently the filler port is removed; this can be done easily under local anaesthesia. If there is any question of post-operative radiotherapy being required after mastectomy, tissue expansion or prosthesis placement is not recommended as the fibrosis consequent to radiotherapy does not allow adequate tissue expansion. Even when fractionation over a longer period is used, capsular contracture affects up to half of patients with implants or tissue expanders following radiotherapy.

To achieve symmetry, it is often necessary to perform a reduction or a mastopexy on the opposite breast, particularly when tissue expanders are used (Figure 25.6). It is important that other possible operations are discussed with the patient at the outset and then they have a realistic view of the likely cosmetic result. All units performing breast reconstruction should provide a photograph album of likely results and patients should be given the opportunity of meeting and discussing the procedure with other patients who have previously undergone the same operation.

Infection of a tissue expander/prosthesis occurs in up to 5% of patients and almost invariably results in the device having to be removed. In order to prevent this disaster, most units use prophylactic antibiotics.

The patient opts to have tamoxifen therapy alone and returns 6 months later complaining of problems related to the tamoxifen. Specifically, she has vaginal dryness and repeated hot flushings which are interfering with the quality of her life. How should these symptoms be treated?

Simple creams such as Replens can improve vaginal dryness. If this fails, local oestrogen preparations which are associated with a low rate of systemic absorption, such as oestradiol given as vaginal tablets (Vagifem), are usually successful in improving the vaginal dryness which occurs as a consequence of the anti-oestrogenic activity of tamoxifen. Hot flushes, as they are known in the UK, or hot flashes, as they are called in the USA, can be improved by the use of progestogens. Megestrol acetate in a dose of 20 mg twice daily is effective in just over half of women and can be combined with tamoxifen. Patients should be warned that, in the first few days after treatment, the frequency of hot flushes/flashes will increase and thereafter, if the drug is effective, they should decrease in frequency. Providing symptoms improve, the dose of megestrol acetate can be reduced by trial and error to the minimum dose that is effective in controlling the symptoms. This is to avoid the side effect of weight gain, which is the most frequent and distressing side effect of this drug. The other agent which has proven effectiveness in this situation is soya, although this has to be delivered in high dose and taken daily. Neither clonidine nor evening primrose oil, which have been tried for this condition, have been shown to be effective in randomized studies.

The patient returns 3 months later and her vaginal dryness has improved but her hot flushes persist despite the megestrol acetate and she states that her quality of life is poor. What options are available for this patient?

One option is to reduce the dose of tamoxifen to 10 mg once a day. It is quite clear that a single dose of 20 mg produces a wide range of plasma levels in patients and these levels appear to be related to body mass index. Tamoxifen given in a dose of 10 mg once a day in a patient with a low body mass index may therefore produce adequate therapeutic levels of drug without side effects. As tamoxifen has a long half-life, dividing the 20 mg dose to 10 mg twice a day has no scientific basis.

If this patient's symptoms persist despite a reduced tamoxifen dose, what other options are available?

This patient could be offered hormone replacement therapy. There are no prospective studies looking at the effects of HRT and recurrence. Small series have been published of women taking a combination of tamoxifen and HRT, and showing improvement in menopausal symptoms. There would obviously be concern about giving this patient oestrogen when she has oestrogen receptor-positive breast cancer, but in the presence of debilitating symptoms, low-dose HRT (if she has not had a hysterectomy) or oestrogen replacement alone (if she has had a hysterectomy) could be tried after discussion of the advantages and disadvantages with the patient. It is not clear whether some of the newer agents such as Tibolone, which are gonadomimetic agents and are effective in reducing vasomotor symptoms associated with the menopause, are safer than oestrogens in this situation.

If she did take hormone replacement therapy and her symptoms responded, then this should be given for as short a duration as necessary to control symptoms.

How would treatment have differed if the tumour had been hormone receptor-negative and she had proceeded to mastectomy, with the pathology showing a 3.5 cm grade III cancer with histological evidence of lymphatic/vascular invasion and involvement of 4 of 21 axillary lymph nodes?

She would now fall into the high-risk group for systemic recurrence and treatment should be chemotherapy (probably six cycles of CMF). The expected benefit in a 58-year-old post-menopausal woman would be an annual odds reduction in any event of about 37% and an annual odds of reduction of death of 11% (Table 25.4). The only other question would be whether she should be given tamoxifen in addition to chemotherapy. Current data suggest there are some advantages of tamoxifen in some postmenopausal, oestrogen receptor-negative patients, although it is not clear whether this is a real effect or whether in the current studies patients who had oestrogen receptor-positive tumours were misclassified because of the fact that the portion of tissue removed at the time of surgery and submitted for biochemical analysis did not contain tumour.

Should tamoxifen be given concurrently with chemotherapy or should it be started after the chemotherapy has finished?

There are no clinical data about this but there are some laboratory data to suggest that tamoxifen puts tumour cells into G0 of the growth cycle when they are less sensitive to chemotherapy, so many units only prescribe tamoxifen after the course of chemotherapy has finished.

How long should tamoxifen be taken for?

Current studies suggest the optimal length of treatment is 5 years (Table 25.1). There is no current evidence that taking tamoxifen for more prolonged periods is advantageous.

What are the potential detrimental effects of tamoxifen?

Tamoxifen is known to increase the incidence of carcinoma in the endometrium, but it does decrease the risk of contralateral breast cancers, and the data show a reduction in overall cancer incidence (Table 25.5). Endometrial cancer is, however, rare and is usually superficial at diagnosis. There is no evidence that endometrial screening of these patients is worth while, although it is practised widely in the USA. Transvaginal ultrasound scanning has been used as a method of screening but the problem is that the apparent endometrial thickness as measured on transvaginal ultrasound scanning increases the longer a patient is on tamoxifen (Figure 25.7). When these patients are hysteroscoped, however, there is rarely evidence of endometrial hyperplasia but of cystic change in the endometrium. The problem with transvaginal ultrasound therefore is that there is a high rate of false positives with this test. In the absence

Table 25.5 Effects of treatment on incidence of endometrial cancer and contralateral cancer in randomized controlled trials of tamoxifen

	Tamoxifen	Control
Endometrial cancer incidence	92	32
Contralateral cancer incidence	369	485
Total events	461	517

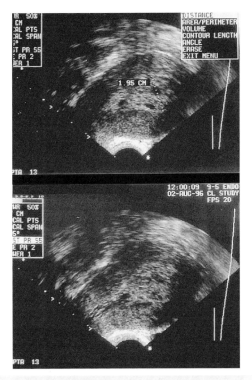

Fig. 25.7 Thickened endometrium on transvaginal ultrasound.

of any appropriate screening test, the current advice is that patients should only be investigated if they have symptoms, the major symptom of endometrial cancer being post-menopausal vaginal bleeding.

26 A 60-year-old woman whose screening mammogram is suspicious

L A Venta and M Morrow

Mrs S is a 60-year-old post-menopausal woman with no clinical breast complaints and no breast cancer risk factors. Her screening mammogram is shown (Figure 26.1). What additional radiologic investigations should be performed?

The screening mammograms shows the breast parenchyma to be composed of mixed fatty and fibroglandular elements. In both upper-outer quadrants there are focal nodular densities, with a suggestion of a spiculated mass in the left (Figure 26.1a and b). The findings on the screening mammogram are inconclusive and warrant further

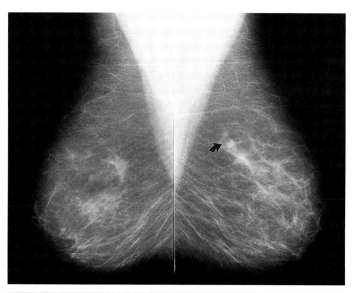

Fig. 26.1(a) Screening mammogram. Mediolateral projection of both breasts demonstrates focal nodular densities with a suggestion of a spiculated mass in the left upper outer quadrant (arrow).

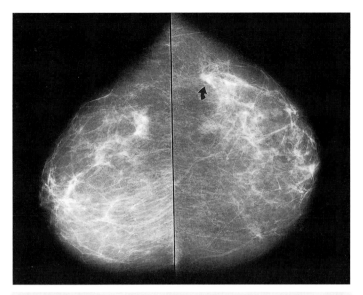

Fig. 26.1(b) Screening mammogram. Craniocaudal projection of both breasts demonstrates focal nodular densities with a suggestion of a spiculated mass in the left upper outer quadrant (arrow).

evaluation. The next step is to evaluate areas of concern with a diagnostic mammogram. A diagnostic mammogram encompasses special projections in an effort to characterize the findings as either normal tissue or a breast mass. The most common projections obtained include spot compression with magnification views of the questionable lesion. If a breast mass is confirmed on these additional views, ultrasound can be used to further characterize it as solid or cystic, and to guide percutaneous biopsy of a suspicious lesion.

A spot compression mammogram confirms the presence of a true mass, and ultrasound demonstrates that it is solid. What are the diagnostic options available to this patient?

Spot compression and magnification of the left upper-outer quadrant in this patient confirms the presence of a small spiculated mass associated with microcalcifications (Figure 26.2). This mammogram appearance is highly suspicious for malignancy and biopsy is indicated. Since this mass is also visible with ultrasound, the patient has several diagnostic options. First, the lesion can be completely excised surgically. Since this is a non-palpable mass, pre-operative needle localization would be required.

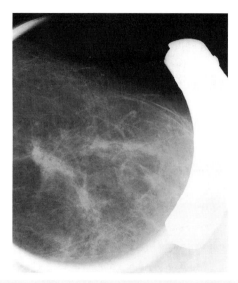

Fig. 26.2 Diagnostic mammogram. Spot compression and magnification view in craniocaudal projection confirms the presence of a mass with spiculated margins and associated microcalcifications.

Alternatively, and preferably, histologic sampling of this lesion can be obtained percutaneously either under mammographic guidance (if stereotactic equipment is available) or with ultrasound guidance. In general, core biopsy with an 11 or 14 gauge needle provides histologic information and is more specific than cytologic aspirates retrieved with fine needles. Both procedures are well tolerated by patients and performed under local anaesthesia. Patients usually prefer ultrasound guidance over stereotactic guidance when given a choice. This is because ultrasound-guided biopsy is performed with the patient supine, the breast is not compressed, and local anaesthesia can be used freely without the risk of obscuring the lesion. Stereotactic biopsy is performed with the patient prone or sitting, the breast being held in compression during the entire procedure and local anaesthesia is used cautiously so as not to obscure the lesion. Thus, stereotactic biopsy is best reserved for patients with either masses not seen by ultrasound or for microcalcifications.

In this patient the decision was made to obtain the diagnosis preoperatively using ultrasound-guided core biopsy. As long as invasive cancer is confirmed histologically on core biopsy, definitive breast cancer resection, be it lumpectomy or mastectomy, and axillary node dissection can both be performed as a single surgical procedure. The disadvantage of this approach is that the histologic diagnosis is based on the core sample and not on the evaluation of the entire lesion. Thus, sampling error must be considered in instances where the histologic diagnosis is discordant with the mammographic findings.

Pre-operative needle localization and excisional biopsy avoids the possibility of sampling errors, as the lesion is removed in its entirety. In patients opting for lumpectomy, the excisional biopsy can also serve as the local breast cancer surgery, if negative margins are achieved. The disadvantage of this approach is that, in almost all cases, the patient will need to undergo a second surgical procedure for axillary lymph node resection and staging.

An ultrasound-guided core biopsy demonstrates infiltrating lobular carcinoma, grade 1 and immunohistochemical oestrogen and progesterone receptors are positive. What are the options for local therapy?

This patient with a small infiltrating lobular carcinoma is an excellent candidate for breast conserving therapy consisting of a lumpectomy, axillary dissection and breast irradiation. Several studies have addressed the question of whether patients with infiltrating lobular carcinoma have a higher risk of local failure in the breast than patients with infiltrating ductal carcinoma, and this does not seem to be the case. The extent of infiltrating lobular carcinoma may be more difficult to determine intra-operatively, owing to its growth pattern of single cells interspersed in the breast stroma. However, provided that negative margins are obtained, local failure rates are similar to those seen with other histologic tumour types, approximately 6-8% at 10 years.

The patient opts for breast conserving therapy, but is concerned about the sequelae of axillary dissection. How common are these problems and could axillary dissection be eliminated in this patient?

Complications of axillary surgery are outlined on page 98. Morbidity includes lymphoedema, numbness in the distribution of the intercostobrachial nerve, decreased range of motion and chronic pain. Axillary dissection in a patient with a grade I small breast cancer in a clinically node-negative axilla should be limited to the level I and II nodes. This procedure identifies nodal metastases with 99% accuracy, since isolated disease at level III in the absence of level I and II node involvement, or skip metastases, is uncommon. The axillary vein should not be stripped, the intercostobrachial nerve should be identified and preserved. With this technique, the complications following a full level III axillary dissection are rare. Since this patient's risk of metastases is relatively low, an axillary node sampling or a level I dissection could be considered. However, clear evidence that a level I dissection reduces morbidity compared to a level I and II dissection is lacking. In contrast, there is evidence that an axillary node sampling is associated with significantly less morbidity than more extensive axillary dissections.

As outlined on page 97, sentinel lymph node biopsy is a new technique in which the first lymph node draining the tumour is identified by injecting the tumour site with blue dye or radiolabelled colloid. If subsequent studies demonstrate its accuracy, this patient would be an ideal candidate for this technique. If she was node negative, she would benefit in terms of reduced morbidity.

Overall, 35% of patients with a clinically negative axilla will have nodal metastases. For tumours less than 1 cm in size, the risk of nodal involvement is between 15% and 20% (Table 26.1). This patient's tumour has favourable prognostic features (low grade, positive receptors) so her risk of nodal disease is low. However, large studies using multiple prognostic factors have been unable to identify

Table 26.1 Frequency of axillary node involvement related to tumour size

Tumour size (cm)	Frequency of axillary node involvement (%)
<0.5	20.6
0.5–0.9	20.6
1–1.9	33.2
2–2.9	44.9
3–3.9	52.1
4–4.9	60.0
>5.0	70.1

From Carter C, Allen C and Henson D. Relation of tumour size, lymph node status and survival in 24,470 breast cancer cases. CANCER, Vol. 63, 1989, p. 181. Copyright © 1989 American Cancer Society. Reprinted by permission of Wiley-Liss, Inc., a subsidiary of John Wiley & Sons, Inc.

Table 26.2 Five-year breast cancer survival rates according to the size of the tumour and axillary node involvement

Tumour size (cm)	Patients surviving 5 years		
	Negative nodes	1–3 positive nodes	Four or more positive nodes
<0.5	269 (99.2%)	53 (95.3%)	17 (59.0%)
0.5–0.9	791 (98.3%)	140 (94.0%)	65 (54.2%)
1–1.9	4668 (95.8%)	1574 (86.6%)	742 (67.2%)
2–2.9	4010 (92.3%)	1897 (83.4%)	1375 (63.4%)
3–3.9	2072 (86.2%)	1185 (79.0%)	1072 (56.9%)
4–4.9	845 (84.6%)	540 (69.8%)	727 (52.6%)
⩾5.0	809 (82.2%)	630 (73.0%)	1259 (45.5%)

From Carter C, Allen C and Henson D. Relation of tumour size, lymph node status and survival in 24,470 breast cancer cases. CANCER, Vol. 63, 1989, p. 181. Copyright © 1989 American Cancer Society. Reprinted by permission of Wiley-Liss, Inc., a subsidiary of John Wiley & Sons, Inc.

reproducibly a subgroup of patients with less than a 10% risk of nodal disease.

The final question about this patient is whether the identification of nodal metastases would alter her therapy and in this case it might. It would certainly alter her survival (Table 26.2). If her tumour is less than 1 cm in size and there is no nodal involvement, she would have over a 98% probability of surviving 5 years and the current view would be that she should not receive adjuvant systemic therapy. If she had 1–3 positive nodes, her 5-year survival would be 94% and she should receive tamoxifen 20 mg daily for 5 years. If more than four positive nodes are identified, then her survival would be dramatically reduced to just over 50% for 5-year survival (Table 26.2) and she would be a candidate for both chemotherapy and tamoxifen.

The patient undergoes lumpectomy and pathology demonstrates a 0.6 cm infiltrating lobular carcinoma which is excised by a minimum of a 1 cm negative margin. Her nodes are negative. Is breast irradiation necessary?

Several randomized studies have addressed the question of whether breast irradiation can be avoided after lumpectomy. The use of irradiation reduces the risk of a breast recurrence by 80–90%. Although breast irradiation does not influence survival, it greatly enhances the patient's chance of preserving her breast and without clinical trials, she should be given radiotherapy.

J M Dixon

A 52-year-old woman has no breast cancer risk factors and no breast complaints. Clinical examination of her breasts is normal. Should she have a screening mammogram?

Screening is the presumptive identification of unrecognized disease by the application of tests, examinations or other procedures which can be applied rapidly. Presumptive is the important word because all screening does is identify two groups of individuals: test positive and test negative. Those who are test positive require a series of diagnostic investigations to determine whether they do truly have the disease being sought whereas those who are test negative should not need to be further investigated. Screening tests should be simple to apply, cheap, easy to perform, easy and unambiguous to interpret, have the ability to define those with disease, and exclude those without disease. Mammography is expensive, requires high-technology equipment, requires special film and processing, needs highly trained radiologists to interpret the films, and detects only 95% of breast cancers at best, and many lesions it identifies are benign. Mammography is, however, the best screening tool available for the detection of breast cancer and is in fact the only screening modality for any malignancy for which the value has been demonstrated by rigorous randomized trials.

A number of randomized trials have been undertaken in Europe and the USA; in addition, there have been a number of non-randomized population-based screening programmes (such as in the UK). There is considerable agreement among trials in showing a reduction in breast cancer mortality between the ages of 50 and 70 (Figure 27.1). For women over the age of 50, trials indicate an average reduction in

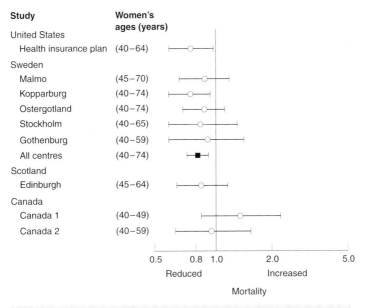

Study	Women's ages (years)
United States	
Health insurance plan	(40–64)
Sweden	
Malmo	(45–70)
Kopparburg	(40–74)
Ostergotland	(40–74)
Stockholm	(40–65)
Gothenburg	(40–59)
All centres	(40–74)
Scotland	
Edinburgh	(45–64)
Canada	
Canada 1	(40–49)
Canada 2	(40–59)

0.5   0.8 1.0   2.0   5.0

Reduced   Increased

Mortality

Fig. 27.1 Summary of 7–12 years' mortality data from randomized trials of breast cancer screening. Points and lines represent absolute change in mortality and confidence interval. (From: Dixon JM. ABC of Breast Diseases. London: BMJ Publishing Group 1995; p. 22, with permission.)

mortality of 29%. If one actually estimates the reduction of mortality in those who attend for screening, then it is estimated that 40% of breast cancer deaths in attenders can be delayed or prevented. This translates into a 1–2% reduction in overall mortality for women over the age of 50 years. Compliance, that is the percentage of those invited for screening who attend, is a major factor influencing the effectiveness of screening and, as compliance falls, so do the benefits of screening.

When compared with patients with symptomatic cancers, breast carcinomas detected by screening are more likely to be small and non-invasive rather than invasive, and those invasive cancers that are detected are more likely to be better differentiated and of special type. Screen-detected cancers are more likely to be node-negative than symptomatic cancers of the same size. The ability of screening to detect cancers at an early stage and to influence subsequent mortality indicates that screening must be detecting small breast cancers before they have the ability to develop metastatic disease.

Some well-differentiated invasive cancers and a number of *in situ* cancers would almost certainly not have caused symptoms during the patient's lifetime. There are no indications from the currently available data that invasive breast carcinomas are being overdiagnosed by screening. It is possible a number of cases of *in situ* carcinoma are detected by screening which would not become clinically significant and some of these individuals may receive unnecessary treatment. Until more is known of the natural history of the type of carcinoma *in situ* detected by screening, the extent to which overdiagnosis and overtreatment actually occurs during screening programmes will remain unknown.

Great debate as to the benefits of screening women in the 40–50 year age group is ongoing. Although breast cancer incidence is substantially higher when all women over 50 are considered, the incidence in a woman aged 45 is 1.6 per 1000 compared to 2.5 per 1000 for a 55-year-old woman. A meta-analysis of population-based screening trials has demonstrated a 24% reduction in breast cancer mortality in women aged younger than 50.

Screening benefits in younger women have been more difficult to detect, owing to the longer screening intervals used in many trials designed to study screening in older women. Evidence indicates that lead time is shorter in younger women and maximum benefits of screening have been seen in the studies with one-year intervals between mammograms. The cost effectiveness of this approach is a subject of debate and ongoing study.

The most appropriate interval between mammographic screens has yet to be determined. Although from a cost–benefit point of view (cost per year of life gained and cost of quality-adjusted year of life saved), 3-yearly screening of women aged 50–64 years of age appears to be the most cost-effective screening policy, the interval cancer rate climbs rapidly between the second and third year after the initial screen, suggesting that this 3-year interval is too long (Figure 27.1). Both annual screening and screening every 2 years have shown comparable survival benefits.

Studies have indicated that all patients should have two views at the first screen. Debate continues on how many views they should have at subsequent screens but, although most units in the UK screen on the second and subsequent occasions with a single view, in the USA, two-view screening is the norm on all visits. There is no evidence that screening using clinical examination, breast ultrasound or teaching patients to perform regular breast self-examination are effective tools at reducing breast cancer mortality. There is some evidence that women who perform regular breast self-examination do detect smaller tumours than those who do not. The problem with breast self-examination is that it needs to be taught by experienced personnel and this is costly. Furthermore, only 30–50% of women who are invited to be taught breast self-examination attend and little is known of the extent to which women comply and continue to practise breast self-examination thereafter. Those studies which have relied on breast self-examination as a screening tool have failed to demonstrate a consistent and significant reduction in mortality in those women invited to be taught breast self-examination. There are also concerns that regular breast self-examination induces anxiety among women who practise it, and this may result in an increased rate of referral to hospital and an increase in the number of benign breast masses detected. While women should be encouraged to examine their own breasts and get to know their 'lumps and bumps', it is not worthwhile investing money in teaching women regular breast self-examination.

The woman has a mammogram and an area of distortion is visualized (Figure 27.2). What are the features and the possible diagnosis?

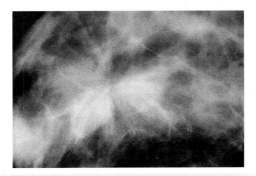

Fig. 27.2 Mammogram showing a radial scar.

Mammographically this patient has a stellate lesion in the breast, which could either be a benign scarring lesion, either a radial scar, a complex sclerosing lesion or sclerosing adenosis, or she could have a small cancer.

How should she be investigated?

This patient should have an image-guided fine-needle aspirate or preferably an image-guided core biopsy.

The core biopsies are obtained and suggest the lesion is benign. Is any further investigation necessary?

Although it has been reported that core biopsy can accurately diagnose scar lesions, it is routine in most centres to remove these stellate lesions to assess the whole lesion. Magnetic resonance imaging has been reported to be of value in differentiating between areas of scarring and small breast cancers.

This patient had the lesion removed and the lesion causing the mammographic abnormality was a radial scar. What is a radial scar?

During involution, areas of excessive scarring can produce stellate lesions which mammographically mimic those of breast cancer. Pathologically these sclerosing lesions can be separated into three groups: sclerosing adenosis, radial scars and complex sclerosing lesions (this term incorporates lesions previously called sclerosing papillomatosis or duct adenoma, and includes infiltrating epitheliosis). There remains doubt as to whether a definitive diagnosis can be made on core biopsy. The reason is that many radial scars or complex sclerosing lesions contain small areas of epithelial proliferation. The frequency with which some of these lesions are associated with tubular cancers is such that some have suggested that they are risk lesions for breast cancer. Excision biopsy is usually required to make a definitive diagnosis.

Do women on hormone replacement therapy require screening starting at an earlier age or more frequent screening than that offered to other women?

The consensus view is that women do not require mammography prior to starting HRT, although all women should have a full clinical examination before HRT is instituted. Most women on HRT are within the age ranges of current screening programmes. HRT does increase the density of the breast and therefore potentially lowers the sensitivity of mammography as a screening tool in these women (Figure 27.3).

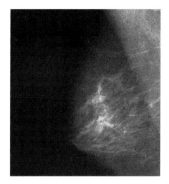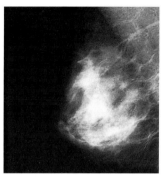

Fig. 27.3 Effects of HRT on the mammographic appearance of the breast. Left, Before starting HRT; right, 3 years after commencing HRT.

28 A 34-year-old woman presents with a short history of a diffusely swollen, red and tender breast

J M Dixon and R C F Leonard

A 34-year-old attends with the complaint that her right breast is diffusely swollen, red and tender (Figure 28.1, see colour plate also). On examination there is no obvious localized mass, but there is *peau d'orange* and erythema of most of the skin of the breast and there are palpable nodes in the axilla. Her doctor telephones for advice, what would you suggest?

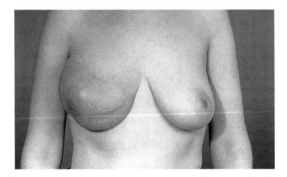

Fig. 28.1 Inflammatory cancer affecting the right breast.

As it can be difficult to differentiate between breast infection and inflammatory cancer, it is appropriate to suggest giving the patient antibiotics and arranging an urgent hospital referral. Inflammatory cancers of the breast can present as a diffusely swollen breast without a localized mass lesion and this can make the diagnosis difficult in some patients. *Peau d'orange* is, however, fairly characteristic of an inflammatory cancer, although it is occasionally seen in infection. Regional nodes should be examined and, if they are pathologically enlarged and clinically suspicious, then it does make malignancy more likely.

When seen in hospital, no localized mass lesion is palpable, the mammograms show diffuse breast oedema but no localized abnormality, and ultrasound shows a diffusely abnormal breast parenchyma but no localized lesion. What would you do next?

There are a number of alternatives. The first would be to assess the axillary nodes and, if these are clinically malignant, then a definitive diagnosis might be obtained by performing cytology or biopsy of the axillary nodes. Alternatively, fine-needle aspiration cytology or preferably core biopsies could be obtained from the areas in the breast of maximum induration to establish a diagnosis. If both of these fail, then an open biopsy of the areas of maximum induration incorporating a portion of overlying skin may confirm the clinical diagnosis. The classic features of an inflammatory cancer are malignant cells visible in lymphatic channels immediately below the skin. As inflammatory cancers are usually treated by primary systemic therapy, it is important to establish a histological diagnosis prior to starting treatment.

Inflammatory breast cancer is one type of locally advanced breast cancer (LABC) (Table 28.1). LABC may arise because of position in the breast (for example, the cancer is peripheral or superficial), neglect (some patients do not present to hospital for months or years after they notice a mass) or biological aggressiveness (this includes all inflammatory cancers and most with *peau d'orange*). Inflammatory carcinomas are uncommon and are characterized by brawny oedematous indurated erythematous skin changes and have the worst

Table 28.1 Clinical features of locally advanced breast disease

Skin
- Ulceration
- Dermal infiltration
- Erythema over tumour
- Satellite nodules
- *Peau d'orange*

Chest wall
- Ribs
- Serratus anterior
- Intercostal muscles

Axillary nodes
- Nodes fixed to one another or to other structures

Table 28.2 Outcome with mastectomy alone in locally advanced breast cancer

Clinical finding	% local recurrence	% 5-year survival
Extensive *peau d'orange*	61	0
Satellite nodules	57	0
Inflammatory cancer	60	0
Ulceration	22	18

prognosis of all LABCs. Studies have shown that a combination of local and systemic therapy produces significant improvements in the control of local disease on the chest wall, and it appears that primary (neo-adjuvant) chemotherapy also has an effect on metastatic progression. Local and regional relapse is a major problem in LABC and affects more than half of patients.

Historically, patients with LABC were treated with a radical mastectomy whenever possible but the results were poor (Table 28.2). The clinical features that correlated with poor outcome were extensive *peau d'orange*, satellite nodules, inflammatory cancers and ulceration (Table 28.1). Subsequently, these patients were treated primarily with radiation therapy alone or radiation therapy followed by surgery, but the prognosis did not improve. Subsequent introduction of effective neo-adjuvant chemotherapeutic regimes (Table 28.3) has improved local control rates and has also had an effect on survival rates. The use of primary chemotherapy reduces tumour size and converts many cases of inoperable breast cancer to operable. Theoretically, the chemotherapy should also help eradicate micrometastatic disease.

Table 28.3 Summary of studies and response rate using different chemotherapeutic regimens used in locally advanced breast cancer

Chemotherapy regimen	Number of studies	Number of courses	Number of patients	% response rate	% complete responses
FAC	7	2–4	576	31–87	8–30
Other Adriamycin regimen	13	2–11	1506	50–91	2–52
CMF	2	3–4	139	47–70	8
Mitomycin regimens	2	4	114	51–94	7–44

FAC, methotrexate/5-fluorouracil; CMF, cytophosphamide.

A histological diagnosis of breast cancer is obtained. How should this young woman with what is clinically an inflammatory breast cancer be treated?

Having established a histological diagnosis of invasive breast cancer, the initial treatment would be chemotherapy. There have been no direct comparisons between different chemotherapy regimes. Generally, there is a high rate of response (Table 28.3). Some recent data suggest that infusional treatment with 5-fluorouracil combined with the anthracyclines, doxorubicin or epirubicin, in regimens with cyclophosphamide or cisplatin produce higher response rates than intermittent regimens, which have been used in this disease setting. Currently 4–6 cycles of treatment are given and further treatment depends on the response. Response rates vary in different series (Table 28.3). Complete clinical response rates of between 30% and 40% have been recorded, although the rate of complete response as assessed histologically is much lower at between 10% and 15%.

The effects of using chemotherapy as initial treatment followed by radiation therapy and surgery are not clear. Of the data that are available (Table 28.4) combinations of chemotherapy, surgery and radiotherapy give the best local control rates. Of 171 women with LABC, treated at the MD Anderson with 3–4 cycles of neo-adjuvant chemotherapy, the objective response rate was 87% and the complete response rate was 10%. Neo-adjuvant chemotherapy appeared to improve disease-free and overall survival rates compared with historical controls. In stage IIIa disease (see Table 22.5a), the median disease-free interval and overall survival was 102 and 104 months, respectively, in patients treated with surgery and radiation therapy only, whereas the median survival had not been reached at 200 months

Table 28.4 Results of combined modality therapy for inflammatory breast cancer

Therapy	Number of studies	Number of patients	% complete response	Median survival (months)	% alive at 3 years (range)	% alive at 5 years (range)
HT	2	2	N/A	12–22	25	0–7
XRT + HT	3	14	N/A	< 12–22	10	0
S + HT ± XRT	13	13	N/A	< 12	0	0

HT, hormonal therapy; XRT, radiotherapy; S, surgery.

in patients treated with neo-adjuvant chemotherapy followed by surgery and/or radiotherapy. In stage IIIb patients (see Table 22.5a), the differences in both disease-free and overall survival were 10 survival points better when combinations of chemotherapy, surgery and radiotherapy were compared with historical controls.

Is conservation therapy possible following chemotherapy in these patients?

For those who respond well to chemotherapy, studies have shown that, if the disease becomes operable and localized, wide local excision followed by post-operative radiotherapy can produce satisfactory local control rates (Table 28.5). Standard therapy for patients whose disease become operable after chemotherapy is mastectomy followed by post-operative radiotherapy. Post-operative adjuvant chemotherapy usually follows surgery, the regimen depending on the pathological assessment of response to initial chemotherapy. For a tumour which is oestrogen receptor-positive as assessed on the initial biopsy, post-operative therapy would include a combination of chemotherapy and hormonal therapy, which in pre-menopausal women is usually tamoxifen or ovarian ablation. For patients whose tumour does not respond or whose tumour becomes smaller but still show signs of local advancement (the inflammation and *peau d'orange* do not disappear), radiotherapy is given to the breast, axilla and supraclavicular fossa in a dose of 40–50 Gy over 15–25 fractions during a 3–5-week period (Figure 28.2). This can be accompanied by a boost to the tumour mass given by external beam or radioactive implant at a dose of 10–20 Gy.

Table 28.5 Results of induction chemotherapy followed by breast conservation in locally advanced breast cancer: summary of data on 189 women with locally advanced breast cancer (30 with inflammatory disease) from Schwartz *et al.* (1994). Induction chemotherapy followed by breast conservation for locally advanced cancer of the breast. CANCER, Vol. 73, p. 362.*

Operation	Number of patients	Number of patients with isolated local recurrences	%
Mastectomy	103	4	4
Wide local excision	55	1	2

*Response rate was 85% allowing 158 patients to have surgery.

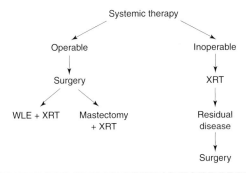

Fig. 28.2 Flow diagram of how to treat inflammatory breast cancer.

Table 28.6 Radiotherapy for locally advanced breast cancer

Treatment areas
- Breast
- Axilla and supraclavicular fossa

Treatment
- Megavoltage X-rays
- Technique for enhancing skin dose
- 40–50 Gy in 15–25 fractions over 3–5 weeks
- Boost to tumour mass if possible by external beam or radioactive implant of 10–20 Gy

Toxicity
- Lethargy
- Skin erythema and small areas of moist desquamation
- Temporary mild dysphagia
- <3% risk of pneumonitis

The breast skin requires full dose, which can produce temporary erythema and desquamation (Table 28.6).

What chemotherapy should be given after surgery or radiotherapy?

Post-operative adjuvant chemotherapy is usually given after surgery or radiotherapy, the regimen depending on the pathological assessment of the response to initial chemotherapy. There is only one randomized clinical trial that has addressed the issue of the need and usefulness of 'adjuvant' chemotherapy following pre-operative or pre-radiotherapy treatment (De Lena *et al.*, 1978 – see Further Reading). In this trial, after three cycles of primary chemotherapy and radiotherapy, the administration of six cycles of additional treatment prolonged both progression-free and overall survival. In early breast cancer, the trend in adjuvant chemotherapy has been to use a single regimen of chemotherapy and to reduce the duration of chemotherapy to between 4 and 6 cycles. This may be optimal for locally advanced breast cancer too, although no definitive data exist. The current trend in clinical trials is to introduce a second, presumed non-cross-resistant regimen following primary chemotherapy in an attempt to eradicate resistant tumour cells which remain following the first combination regimen. This is in part the reasoning for using combinations of chemotherapy and hormone therapy.

A 75-year-old woman presents with a 3-year history of a breast lump with overlying ulceration

J M Dixon

A 75-year-old woman presents with a history of a lump in her breast for 3 years which has more recently ulcerated (Figure 29.1, see colour plate also). What is the diagnosis and how should she be treated?

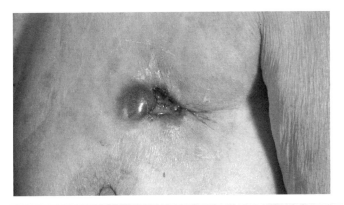

Fig. 29.1 Ulcerated locally advanced breast cancer.

This is a locally advanced breast cancer. Part of the reason it is locally advanced is because of neglect and because the lesion has been present for a long time.

How would you treat this woman?

Fortunately, these tumours tend to be oestrogen receptor-positive. Providing the tumour is confirmed to be oestrogen receptor-positive, she should be treated with an initial 3–6 month course of tamoxifen. This can result in significant responses in up to three-quarters of women and allows some locally advanced breast cancers to become

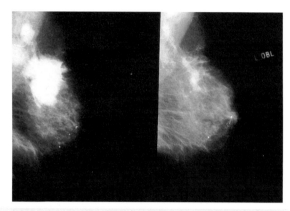

Fig. 29.2 Locally advanced breast cancer before (left) and after 3 months of tamoxifen treatment (right). The tumour has now become operable.

operable and suitable for surgery (Figure 29.2). If surgery is performed, it should be followed by post-operative radiotherapy.

If there is a significant problem with bleeding from the surface of the tumour, then radiotherapy is indicated. If the initial tumour was oestrogen receptor-negative, then the initial treatment should be radiotherapy.

Toilet mastectomy for locally advanced breast cancer is not to be encouraged and is only indicated in patients with localized indolent disease. It should not be performed in patients with multiple satellite nodules and widespread areas of *peau d'orange* where recurrence rates are very high. For some patients with malodorous disease as in this patient, surgical debridement is indicated to reduce malodour.

She is treated with tamoxifen and part of the area of skin ulceration re-epithelializes. She is maintained on tamoxifen therapy for 3 years when she presents to the clinic with a history of increasing breathlessness and a chest X-ray demonstrates a pleural effusion. How common is this and how should she be treated?

Of those patients who develop metastases, up to half will develop a malignant pleural effusion, although only some of these will require specific treatment. Although the fluid can be aspirated to obtain a diagnosis, simple aspiration is not an effective treatment. When interpreting cytology reports, it is important to know that, in only 85% of patients with malignant pleural effusion, will there be malignant cells identified on cytology. For patients with a large pleural effusion, tube drainage followed by a new or changed systemic therapy controls effusions in just over a third of patients. In the other two-thirds who develop recurrent effusions, instillation of tetracycline, bleomycin or occasionally talc is required to control recurrence. When using these agents, the pleural fluid should be aspirated to complete dryness and a small amount of local anaesthetic placed into the pleural cavity before adding the active agent, as this reduces the pain associated with this procedure. Patients who have tetracycline, bleomycin or talc inserted into the pleural cavity often develop a transient pyrexia following this procedure.

The fluid should be drained to dryness and pleurodesis considered. Disease extent should be assessed with a bone scan and an assessment of the liver. In the absence of any life-threatening disease, second line hormone therapy should be instituted and the choice is between the two new aromatase inhibitors, anastrozole 1 mg or letrozole 2.5 mg.

30 A 48-year-old presents with a 6-month history of a lump in the left breast and increasingly severe pain in the mid-thoracic region

W Gradishar

A 48-year-old pre-menopausal woman presents with a 6-month history of a left breast mass which has been increasing in size. For the past month she has had increasingly severe pain in the mid-thoracic region which keeps her from sleeping and is not relieved with over-the-counter analgesics. On physical examination, a 4 cm irregular mass is palpable in the lower outer quadrant of the left breast. Several hard, non-fixed 1 cm axillary nodes are present. There is no supraclavicular adenopathy. A needle biopsy confirms the diagnosis of infiltrating ductal carcinoma, grade III. Hormone receptors are positive. What additional investigations are indicated?

The patient presents with a large primary tumour and several suspicious, enlarged axillary lymph nodes. In addition, the history of severe, unrelenting back pain is suspicious for metastatic disease and raises the concern for an impending spinal cord compression (SCC). The physical examination should be performed with special attention aimed at detecting subtle neurological deficits or point tenderness over the spine. To evaluate the extent of disease the following tests should be performed: full blood count, urea and electrolytes, liver function tests and alkaline phosphatase, chest X-ray, and bone scan. Assessment of the liver by an ultrasound scan or computerized tomography would also be helpful. Any further diagnostic tests should be organized once the results of these initial investigations are available.

A bone scan reveals multiple areas of uptake in the thoracic and lumbar spine and the ribs. Chest X-ray and CT scan of the abdomen

and pelvis are normal. What systemic therapy should the patient receive?

The patient has confirmed metastatic bone disease and the presenting complaints of severe back pain warrant further evaluation to rule out spinal cord compression (SCC). More than 90% of patients who develop SCC from cancer have back pain. If SCC is suspected, then investigations should be directed at excluding this complication while at the same time relieving symptoms. An emergency magnetic resonance imaging or CT myelogram should be obtained. Following one of these investigations, the patient should be assessed by a multidisciplinary team, which should include the opinion of an oncologist, a radiotherapist, and an orthopaedic surgeon or a neurosurgeon with a special interest in spinal disease.

What should be done to control the patient's back pain?

If the evaluation does not reveal SCC, then palliative radiotherapy should be considered for the most symptomatic sites in the spine. Bisphosphonate therapy (pamidronate) should also be considered since it has been shown to decrease the morbidity related to lytic bone disease (pain scores, fractures, SCC, etc.). Systemic therapy with chemotherapy or endocrine therapy would also be expected to palliate symptoms, although cure of the disease is unlikely. Several different chemotherapy regimens could be considered in this situation including AC, CMF or doxorubicin/taxoid combinations. This patient could also be considered for treatment with high-dose chemotherapy, but the efficacy of this approach needs to be defined by randomized trials comparing it with standard-dose chemotherapy. Since the tumour is hormone receptor-positive, tamoxifen should be given as part of the treatment.

Would the choice of therapy differ if the patient presented initially with lung or liver metastases?

If the patient had sites of metastases primarily in the lung or liver, then it would be more likely that you would give this patient systemic chemotherapy alone, or a combination of chemotherapy and hormonal therapy (i.e. tamoxifen). The chemotherapy treatment options would be identical to those outlined above. If significant tumour shrinkage was observed, then investigational approaches using high-dose chemotherapy and peripheral stem transplantation could be considered, but the likelihood of curing the disease is low.

During the course of her metastatic work-up, the patient experiences difficulty voiding and numbness in her legs. What evaluation and therapy is indicated?

The symptoms described raise the concern of an impending SCC. If the diagnostic evaluation confirms SCC, then intravenous dexamethasone should be administered (10 mg initially, followed by 4-6 mg every 6 hours) to decrease peritumoural oedema, which may develop in association with SCC. A dramatic improvement in both symptoms and clinical findings is often observed immediately after the administration of steroids. An emergency neurosurgical and radiation therapy consultation should be obtained. The goal of intervention is to preserve neurological function. In the patient described, bladder function and sensory function are already impaired. The greater the neurological deficit at presentation, the less likely *any* intervention is to correct the deficit. Two approaches are considered in this setting. Radiation therapy can be directed to the area of SCC. If significant spinal disease is present, a back brace may be required for support during any type of significant movement or ambulating. The other approach is surgical and involves a decompression laminectomy in the area of SCC. The affected vertebral body or a portion of it is removed, and the area is supported with rods and/or surgical cement. The studies that have compared outcomes between radiotherapy and laminectomy have been cited as demonstrating that spinal surgery has a small role to play in the management of SCC. Laminectomy alone, however, is not the operative treatment of choice in a modern setting in patients with SCC. With modern imaging and surgical instrumentation, it is possible to decompress and stabilize the vertebral column either anteriorly or posteriorly to an extent which was generally not possible at the time during which these largely retrospective and unrandomized studies were reported. It is probable in the absence of more modern studies that surgical decompression and stabilization combined with post-operative radiotherapy offers the best quality of life for many of these patients. When surgical intervention is undertaken, the use of MRI-compatible fixators is recommended as this greatly facilitates future assessment.

Radiotherapy should be given if surgical decompression is not appropriate and this should be given in a number of fractions.

For patients who have already received radiation to the area of SCC, decompressive surgery is the treatment of choice if they develop further symptoms.

One year after receiving chemotherapy and irradiation for the treatment of bone metastases, the patient is asymptomatic and re-staging work-up reveals no new sites of metastases. Is local therapy of the breast indicated?

Although the patient has stable disease, she will not be cured of metastatic breast cancer. If the breast lesion remains stable and asymptomatic, then no further local therapy is indicated. However, if the breast lesion is causing symptoms (i.e. pain, skin breakdown, discharge), a mastectomy or local radiation therapy could be considered. It is important to recognize that the disease that will dictate survival is not located in the breast but rather at sites of distant metastases.

A 45-year-old woman presents having noticed an enlarged axillary node

J M Dixon

A 45-year-old woman attends having noticed an enlarged axillary node. Clinically, when you examine her there is a 2 cm fairly discrete node in the axilla which you consider pathological but no breast mass is present. What are the possible causes and how do you investigate her?

A lesion of this size is likely to be malignant and to represent either metastatic involvement of a node or a primary lymphoma. Very occasionally such large nodes can be benign and are seen in association with systemic disorders such as rheumatoid arthritis, sarcoid or even tuberculosis. A complete history should be taken and a full examination performed including assessment of other regional nodes.

How would you investigate this patient?

This patient should have a mammogram which may show the abnormal node (Figure 31.1) and may identify a cause for the mass. The next investigation should be a fine-needle aspirate or core biopsy. On cytology, it is usually, but not always, possible to differentiate a lymphoma from metastatic cancer. A core biopsy has the advantage that it can reliably differentiate between lymphoma and metastatic breast cancer because it allows tumour marker studies to be performed. If lymphoma is considered likely on cytology, then the node should be excised to obtain a detailed pathological assessment as this will influence treatment.

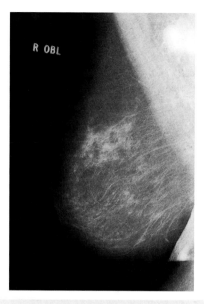

Fig. 31.1 Mammogram of a patient with a breast cancer and an involved axillary node.

Investigations demonstrate this patient has metastatic carcinoma in the axillary nodes but there is no mammographic lesion. How should this patient be further assessed and treated?

Up to 70% of women shown histologically to have metastatic carcinoma in the axillary nodes will have an occult breast cancer; most of these are visible on mammography, ultrasonography or breast magnetic resonance imaging. This patient should, therefore, have a breast ultrasound and if this shows no abnormality a breast MRI and, if a lesion is identified on either of these investigations, then this should be sampled to obtain a cytological or histological diagnosis. It is now possible to localize lesions visible only on MRI. It is also possible sometimes to see MRI visible lesions using high-resolution ultrasound. Other possible primary sites should be considered, particularly lung. All patients require a chest X-ray and, if there is any abnormality on this, then computerized tomography or MRI of the thorax should be performed. If an abnormality is identified on the mammogram, then this should be investigated by image-guided fine-needle aspiration and/ or core biopsy. If carcinoma is confirmed, then this patient should be treated as for any other patient with a breast cancer and involved nodes. Where no lesion is identified and metastatic carcinoma is present in the node, then an axillary dissection should be performed as the first procedure. If metastatic carcinoma is confirmed on the excision specimen and the histology is in keeping with an origin in the breast (features which suggest this histologically include the presence of oestrogen receptors in a tumour which is S100-negative and cytokeratin-positive), then patients should be given the same systemic therapy as that administered to any other women of the same age and disease stage. From the node it is possible to gain some information on tumour grade and oestrogen receptor status.

There are three main options with regard to treating the breast. One is to keep the breast under regular observation and to treat any lesion which appears. This is not a commonly adopted option. The second is to irradiate the breast prophylactically. This approach is thought to be associated with a higher rate of local failure than that seen after partial mastectomy and radiotherapy, owing to the fact that occult tumours can be quite diffuse and it is not possible to deliver a boost to the site of the primary tumour. The third option is to perform a mastectomy with the presumption that the nodal disease is due to a breast primary. With the availability of high-quality mammography, MRI and ultrasound, the rationale for this approach is less compelling. All three approaches have been used in different centres, and reported to be associated with reasonable local control rates and similar survival rates to other patients with involved nodes. In about a third of patients treated by observation, a cancer becomes obvious during follow up, and is then treated either by mastectomy or wide local excision with radiotherapy to the breast.

A 65-year-old woman presents 10 years after mastectomy with a nodule in her mastectomy scar

J M Dixon and R C F Leonard

A 65-year-old woman presents 10 years after mastectomy and axillary node dissection with a nodule in her mastectomy scar. She originally presented with a 4.5 cm breast cancer which was grade II and node-negative. She received no adjuvant systemic therapy at that time and did not receive post-operative radiotherapy. Full staging demonstrates no evidence of metastases. How would you treat her?

Local recurrence after mastectomy usually occurs in the skin flaps adjacent to the scar and is presumed to arise from viable cells shed during surgery. In some patients the disease develops in breast tissue left behind on the mastectomy flaps. Recurrence can usually be diagnosed by fine-needle aspiration cytology. Although local chest wall recurrence can be isolated, in up to half of patients it heralds systemic relapse and it is for this reason that a search for distant metastases should be undertaken in all patients. Local recurrence after mastectomy can be classified as single-spot relapse, multiple-spot relapse or field change (Figures 32.1–32.3, see colour plates also). Treatment and prognosis differ for these three categories.

If the recurrence is focal and occurs many years after the original surgery, excision alone has been reported to provide adequate local control, although most units would consider introducing or changing systemic therapy. If the recurrence is not single, but is still localized, then options are radiotherapy, if not previously given, or a more radical excision. In widespread recurrence, standard chemotherapy regimens are used but often produce disappointing control rates. Intra-arterial chemotherapy and infusional fluorouracil are also options, and have been reported to be effective in some patients where standard

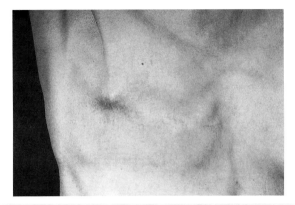

Fig. 32.1 Single spot recurrence after mastectomy.

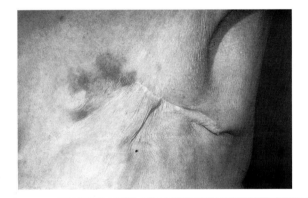

Fig. 32.2 Multiple spot recurrence after mastectomy.

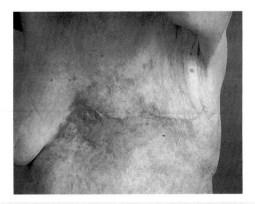

Fig. 32.3 Field recurrence after mastectomy.

approaches have failed. Failure to halt the progress of local disease can lead to cancer *en cuirase*, where the chest wall is encircled by tumour – a most unpleasant situation for the patient.

Recurrence on the chest wall can be quite indolent, grow slowly and occur in the absence of metastases elsewhere. Keeping the disease under control is a considerable problem for both carers and patients. Excision of dead tissue and the use of topical and oral antibiotics with anti-anaerobic activity combined with charcoal dressings help to control the malodour. The best form of treatment is prevention by ensuring that the initial treatment is optimal.

In this patient an excision alone was performed and the lesion was completely excised. What other treatments should she receive?

The options for this patient include giving her radiotherapy to the chest wall or instituting systemic therapy. In part this would depend on the oestrogen receptor result. If she had an oestrogen receptor-positive tumour then a reasonable option would be to start treatment with tamoxifen. If it was oestrogen receptor-negative, then it would be reasonable to consider radiotherapy alone.

The tumour was oestrogen receptor-positive and she was given tamoxifen. The patient should be warned of side effects which, although considered by many to be rare, do occur in over 50% of patients. These include flushings, vaginal dryness or discharge, occasional gastrointestinal upset and weight gain. Treatment should be continuous until the patient develops evidence of progression. This is different from the adjuvant situation where treatment is usually stopped after 5 years.

She presents 4 years later with pain in her right hip. An X-ray shows a lytic lesion in the femur (Figure 32.4). What are the features present and what treatment would you suggest?

There is an obvious lytic lesion in the neck of the femur, which occupies a significant portion of the neck, so there is a danger that a pathological fracture may occur at this site. Optimal treatment for this lesion would be prophylactic total hip replacement (Figure 32.4). After surgery, the area should then be irradiated to ensure long-term local disease control. This patient should also have full staging investigations

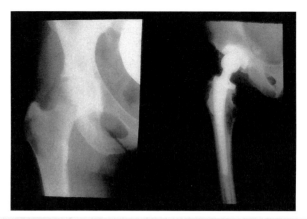

Fig. 32.4 Lytic lesion in the neck of femur before (left) and after total hip replacement (right).

to assess the extent of disease at other sites. Specifically, she should have a chest X-ray, a bone scan and liver ultrasound.

Sixty-five to 70% of patients with breast cancer develop bone metastases. Although the median survival of these patients is only 2 years, 20% of them are alive 5 years later. Approximately half of patients with metastatic breast cancer develop only bone metastases and they die from bone complications.

The bone scan is shown in Figure 32.5. What other investigations would you organize and how would you treat this patient?

The bone scan shows multiple metastases throughout the skeleton. The patient should also have her calcium and phosphate checked to ensure she is not hypercalcaemic. If she has pain at any specific site, then analgesics are the mainstay of treatment in such a patient as a prelude to effective anticancer therapy. Non-steroidal anti-inflammatory drugs are surprisingly potent in dealing with bone pain even when compared with opiates. Combining non-steroidals with opiates increases the efficacy while minimizing side effects. If there were no metastases at other sites, then appropriate treatment would be second-line hormonal therapy with local radiotherapy to any specific sites of particular pain. A single dose of radiotherapy is usually effective for localized bone pain secondary to metastatic disease. Response rates to second-line hormones are in the region of 25–40%. Response to such second-line agents is much more likely

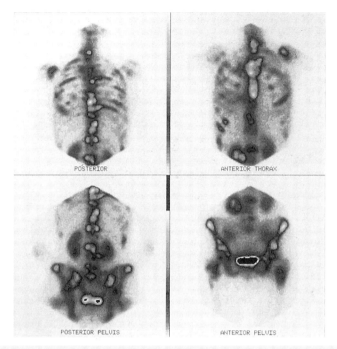

Fig. 32.5 Multiple bone metastases seen on a bone scan.

when there has been a response to first-line hormonal treatment. Options for second-line treatment include the progestogens, megestrol acetate and medroxyprogesterone acetate, and the aromatase inhibitors, lentaron, anastrozole and letrozole. In view of the recent studies, which have shown improvements in response rates and improvements in survival with the new aromatase inhibitors, then the choice is really between anastrozole and letrozole. Both anastrozole and letrozole are highly potent aromatase inhibitors producing between 97% and 99% aromatase inhibition in laboratory tests. The doses are 1 mg of anastrozole and 2.5 mg of letrozole. It is not yet evident whether one has significant advantages over the other. In a study comparing anastrazole versus megestrol acetate, similar response rates were seen but anastrozole (1 mg) produced a significant improvement in overall survival. In a study comparing 2.5 mg of letrozole and megestrol acetate, a significantly higher response rate was seen with letrozole. A second study comparing letrozole with aminoglutethimide has demonstrated a significant survival advantage for 2.5 mg of letrozole over aminoglutethimide.

This patient should also be considered for bisphosphonates. The clinical use of bisphosphonates has increased dramatically during the past five years. Studies have shown that pamidronate reduces the frequency of skeletal events in patients with myeloma or breast cancer by approximately 50%. It is likely that other bisphosphonates will also be shown to be effective. Bisphosphonates inhibit the action of osteoclasts although new studies suggest that the bisphosphonate clodronate may have an effect other than that on osteolysis and bone resorption. Studies suggest that these drugs may decrease the tumour burden in bone and possibly also in soft tissues. The latest study suggests that bisphosphonates can reduce the incidence and number of new bony and visceral metastases in women with breast cancer who are at high risk of distant metastases, and their use in breast cancer is likely to increase.

Measuring the benefit of treatment of bony disease in terms of objective regression of tumour can be difficult with bone scans being unreliable as indicators of response to treatment. If a patient achieves a symptomatic improvement, then this is an indication that the treatment is likely to be working. Tumour markers have been shown to be useful in assessing response in bony disease. CA15–3 in combination with CEA and ESR have been extensively investigated for monitoring therapy. This method of assessment has been confirmed prospectively. Using this combination, all patients are potentially assessable by tumour markers. X-ray assessment of lytic metastases should be undertaken at 3 months and 6 months in the first instance. At 3 months it is recommended that X-rays should be taken of up to two of the key metastases and at 6 months repeat X-rays should be taken of all the key sites.

If she had also had a history of passing increasing amounts of urine and being thirsty. What do you think this patient has developed? What investigations would you perform and how would you treat her if your clinical diagnosis is confirmed?

This patient should have her calcium phosphate and albumin checked because she has clinical symptoms suggestive of hypercalcaemia. Symptomatic hypercalcaemia is usually associated with a serum calcium of > 3 mmol/l. Treatment is by hydration with saline, giving between 3 and 4 l over 24 hours. A single intravenous

infusion of bisphosphonates should be given, either clodronate
1500 mg in 500 ml of saline over 4-6 hours, or pamidronate 15-
90 mg in saline at a maximum infusion rate of 1 mg per minute.
Further effective anti-cancer treatment reduces the risk of recurrence,
but patients whose disease is refractory to this treatment and who
have continued hypercalcaemia can be treated with intravenous
bisphosphonates given every 2-4 weeks. Oral bisphosphonates
(clodronate 1600 mg daily) are available and their role in recurrent
hypercalcaemia is being investigated. Having developed
hypercalcaemia, it is likely that this patient's disease is again
relapsing. Anti-cancer treatment in this patient would probably
consist of third-line hormonal agents which are effective in up to 20%
of patients who respond to first- and second-line drugs. The third-line
agents include megestrol acetate in a dose of 160 mg a day and
medroxyprogesterone acetate in a dose of 500 mg to 1 g daily. The
side effects of these drugs include hirsuitism, weight gain and
breakthrough vaginal bleeding.

33 A 72-year-old man presents with a lump in his left breast which is associated with overlying skin changes

J M Dixon

A 72-year-old presents with a lump in his left breast which is associated with overlying skin changes (Figure 33.1, see colour plate also). What is your clinical diagnosis and how would you investigate him?

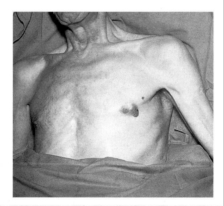

Fig. 33.1 A male with breast cancer.

Clinically there is direct infiltration of the overlying skin by a breast cancer. The investigation of a suspected male breast cancer is identical to that of female breast cancer. The patient should have a full clinical examination for assessment of the mass with regard to its overlying skin involvement, underlying fixation to the underlying muscle and chest wall. The tumour should be carefully measured with callipers and regional nodes assessed. Investigation should include a mammogram (Figure 33.2) and fine-needle aspiration cytology.

Male breast cancer is over 100 times less common than female breast cancer and represents only 0.7% of all cancers which occur in men.

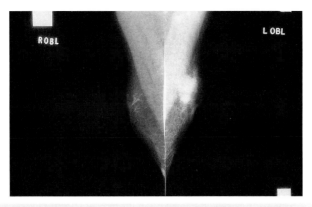

Fig. 33.2 Mammogram of male breast cancer.

One male breast cancer is seen for approximately every 200 female breast cancers and thus represents 0.5% of all breast cancers. The peak age incidence of male breast cancer is 5–10 years older than that in females. The aetiology, like that of female breast cancer, is unknown but there is an increased incidence in patients with Klinefelter syndrome.

How does breast cancer present?

The presenting features are identical to those in females and patients usually present with a lump, skin or nipple retraction and occasionally nipple discharge. Because of the smaller volume of male breasts, male breast cancers are more likely to involve the overlying skin and nipple directly than female breast cancers. The histology of male breast cancer is similar to that in females.

How often do men with breast cancer have a family history?

A family history of breast cancer is present in about 30% of males with breast cancer, and multiple cases of male breast cancer within a family are unusual but have been reported. The most common scenario is that the family contains a number of cases of female breast cancer, and a single or rarely two male breast cancers. The most common cause for such a family history is inheritance of a mutation in the BRCA2 gene on the long arm of chromosome 13.

How should this man be treated?

The historical treatment of choice for male breast cancer has been radical mastectomy. This approach has been advocated because of the concern of achieving complete removal by a modified radical mastectomy. More recently, however, the standard treatment has become modified radical mastectomy and occasional patients are suitable for breast conservation. Adjuvant radiotherapy has been widely used in the treatment of male breast cancer. This improves local control rates, although it has little if any effect on overall survival.

Over 80% of male breast cancers are oestrogen receptor-positive and this is consistent with the finding that, when tamoxifen is used as a first-line treatment in receptor-positive disease, response rates in the range of 50–80% are seen. Although reports have described the benefits of adjuvant chemotherapy, the disease is too uncommon to have allowed randomized trials. Generally, the recommendations regarding selection of adjuvant therapy are similar to those of females with breast cancer. All patients with positive nodes and high-risk node-negative patients should be treated with appropriate systemic therapy.

What are the prognosis and outlook for male breast cancer?

The overall survival of male breast cancer is probably worse than that for women with breast cancer but, when corrected for disease stage, survival is similar. Approximately 30% of men have advanced disease at presentation. For those with node-negative disease, over 80% survive 10 years and this reduces to just over 40% 10-year survival for those with involved nodes.

A 48-year-old woman is treated by breast conservation for breast cancer. During chemotherapy it is clear that she is very anxious and develops signs and symptoms of anxiety and depression

J M Dixon

A 48-year-old is treated by breast conservation. She has involved nodes and is advised to have post-operative radiotherapy and chemotherapy. During her chemotherapy, it is clear that she is very anxious, and develops signs and symptoms of anxiety and depression. How common is this and how should she be treated?

Up to a third of women with breast cancer develop an anxiety state or depressive illness within 1 year of diagnosis. The diagnosis of an anxiety state is based on the criteria set out in Table 34.1. The treatment of an anxiety state depends on how severe it is. For patients finding difficulty coping psychologically, they should be given a benzodiazepine (such as diazepam) on an 'as-needed basis' for up to 3 weeks. This avoids the risk of becoming dependent on this treatment. An alternative would be to prescribe a small dose of a tranquillizer such as thioridizine in a dose of 25 mg three times a day.

Table 34.1 Criteria for anxiety state

- Persistent anxiety, tension or inability to relax
- Present for more than half of the time for 4 weeks
- Cannot pull self out of it or be distracted by others
- Substantial departure from normal mood
- Plus at least four of the following:
  Initial insomnia
  Irritability
  Impaired concentration
  Intolerance of noise
  Panic attacks
  Somatic manifestation like palpitation

Table 34.2 Criteria for depressive illness

- Persistent low mood
- Present for more than half of the time for 4 weeks
- Cannot be distracted out of it by self or others
- Qualitatively or quantitatively significantly different from normal mood
- Inability to enjoy oneself
- Plus at least four of the following:
  Diurnal variation of mood
  Repeated or early waking
  Impaired concentration or indecisiveness
  Feeling hopeless or suicidal
  Feelings of guilt, self-blame, being a burden or worthlessness
  Irritability and anger for no reason
  Loss of interest
  Retardation or agitation

Thereafter, it is worth teaching the techniques for managing anxiety. Any somatic symptoms of anxiety such as palpitations can be treated by using beta-blockers.

The criteria for depressive illness are outlined in Table 34.2. This usually responds well to anti-depressant medication providing it is given in a therapeutic dose and for sufficient time. A correct course is from 4 to 6 months. These drugs do not cause physical dependence. Patients who complain of feeling agitated benefit from a sedating drug such as dothiepin, 75 mg at night, increasing to 150 mg if necessary. Those who are lethargic and apathetic benefit from a more alerting medication, such as fluoxetine, starting at a dose of 20 mg in the morning and increasing to 40 mg if symptoms do not improve. If the anxiety state, depressive illness or other underlying problems persist, then psychiatric referral should be considered.

She vomits profusely during her first course of chemotherapy and thereafter develops anticipatory vomiting prior to her next course of chemotherapy. How common is this and how can it be treated?

Up to a quarter of women given adjuvant chemotherapy develop conditioned responses. Anything that reminds them of the treatment causes them to experience adverse effects such as nausea and vomiting. Thereafter they can become phobic of the hospital or the chemotherapy suite. It is important to do everything possible during the first course of chemotherapy to reduce vomiting by using drugs such as 5-hydroxytryptamine antagonists. Covering each infusion with an anxiolytic drug such as lorazepam 2 mg is also often helpful.

Contents by diagnosis

We recognise that not all readers will wish to refer to the book by symptom. The list below therefore refers to cases by number and diagnosis for ease of reference.

Cases 18 and 19 Nipple Problems

Cases 20–34 Breast Cancer

Further reading

Congenital problems

Supernumerary or accessory nipple/breast

Beals RK, Crawford S. Congenital absence of the pectoral muscles. Clin Orthopaed 1976; 119: 166.

McDowell F. On the propagation, perpetuation and parroting of erroneous eponyms such as 'Poland's syndrome'. Plast Reconstr Surg 1977; 59: 561.

Maliniac JW. Breast Deformities and their Origin. Grune & Stratton, New York, 1950, pp 163.

Osborne MP. Breast development and anatomy. In: Diseases of the Breast. Eds: Harris JR, Lippman ME, Morrow M, Hellman S. Lippincott-Raven, Philadelphia, 1996, pp 1–14.

Pers M. Aplasias of the anterior thoracic wall, the pectoral muscle and the breast. Scand J Plast Reconstr Surg 1968; 2: 125.

Ravitch MM. Poland's syndrome: a study of an eponym. Plast Reconstr Surg 1977; 59: 508.

Simon BE, Hoffman S, Kahn S. Treatment of asymmetry of the breasts. Clinics Plast Surg 1975; 2: 375.

Trier WC. Complete breast absence. Plast Reconstr Surg 1965; 36: 430.

Developmental problems

Breast hypoplasia

Beals RK, Crawford S. Congenital absence of the pectoral muscles. Clin Orthop 1976; 119: 166.

Bostwick J, III. Plastic and Reconstructive Surgery, Volume I. Quality Medical Publishing Inc, St Louis, 1990.

Brown LS, Silverman BG, Berg WA. Rupture of silicone-gel breast implants: causes, sequelae and diagnosis. Lancet 1997; 350: 1531-1537.

Coleman DJ, Foo ITH, Sharpe DT. Textured or smooth implants for breast augmentation: A prospective controlled trial. Br J Plast Surg 1991; 44: 444.

Collis N, Sharpe DT. Breast implant controversy: an update. The Breast 1998; 7: 61-65.

McDowell F. On the propagation, perpetuation and parroting of erroneous eponyms such as 'Poland's syndrome'. Plast Reconstr Surg 1977; 59: 561.

Park AJ, Chetty U, Watson ACH. Silicone breast implants and breast cancer. The Breast 1998; 7: 22-26.

Pers M. Aplasias of the anterior thoracic wall, the anterior muscle, and the breast. Scand J Plast Reconstr Surg 1968; 2: 125.

Peters W, Smith D, Lugowski S. Failure properties of 352 explanted silicone-gel breast implants. Can J Plast Surg 1996; 4: 1.

Ravitch MM. Poland's syndrome: a study of an eponym. Plast Reconstr Surg 1977; 59: 508.

Robinson OG, Bradley EL, Wilson DS. Analysis of explanted silicone implants: a report of 300 patients. Ann Plast Surg 1995; 34: 1-6.

Simon BE, Hoffman S, Kahn S. Treatment of asymmetry of the breasts. Clinics Plast Surg 1975; 2: 375.

Trier WC. Complete breast absence. Plast Reconstr Surg 1965; 36: 430.

Breast hyperplasia – virginal hypertrophy

Bolger WE, Seyfer AE, Jackson SM. Reduction mammaplasty using the inferior glandular 'pyramid' pedicle: experiences with 3000 patients. Plast Reconstr Surg 1987; 80: 75-84.

Bostwick J, III. Plastic and Reconstructive Breast Surgery. Quality Medical Publishing, Inc, St Louis, 1990, pp 293-408.

Lassus C. Breast reduction: evaluation of a technique – a single vertical scar. Aesthet Plast Surg 1987; 11: 107-112.

Lejour M. Vertical Mammaplasty and Liposuction. Quality Medical Publishing, Inc, St Louis, 1994.

Lemperle G, Nievergelt J. Plastic and Reconstructive Breast Surgery: An Atlas. Springer-Verlag, Berlin, 1991.

Robbins TH. A reduction mammaplasty with areola-nipple based on an inferior dermal pedicle. Plast Reconstr Surg 1977; 59: 64-67.

A patient with very small breasts

Asplund O, Gylbert L, Jurell G, Ward C. Textured or smooth implants of submuscular breast augmentation: a controlled study. Plast Reconstr Surg 1995; 97: 1200–1206.

Buckly LP, Ehrlich HP, Sohoni S, May JW. The capsule quality of saline filled smooth saline implants, textured silicone and polyurethane implants in rabbits: a long term study. Plast Reconstr Surg 1994; 93: 1123–1131.

Bostwick J, III. Plastic and Reconstructive Breast Surgery. Quality Medical Publishing, Inc, St Louis, 1990.

Brown LS, Silverman BG, Berg WA. Rupture of silicone-gel breast implants: causes, sequelae and diagnosis. Lancet 1997; 350: 1531–1537.

Coleman DJ, Foo ITH, Sharpe DT. Textured or smooth implants for breast augmentation: A prospective controlled trial. Br J Plast Surg 1991; 44: 444.

Collis N, Sharpe DT. The breast implant controversy: an update. The Breast 1998; 7: 61–65.

La Vier RR, Harrison MC, Cook RR, Lane TH. What is silicone? Plast Reconstr Surg 1993; 92: 163–167.

Lane TH, Burns SA. Silica, silicon and silicones: unravelling the mystery. Curr Top Microbiol Immunol 1996; 210: 3–12.

Park AJ, Chetty U, Watson ACH. Silicone breast implants and breast cancer. The Breast 1998; 7: 22–26.

Peters W, Smith D, Lugowski S. Failure properties of 352 explanted silicone-gel breast implants. Can J Plast Surg 1996; 4: 1.

Robinson OG, Bradley EL, Wilson DS. Analysis of explanted silicone implants: a report of 300 patients. Ann Plast Surg 1995; 34: 1–6.

Gynaecomastia

Algaratnam TT. Idiopathic gynaecomastia treated with tamoxifen: a preliminary report. Clin Ther 1987; 9: 483.

Braunstein GD. Gynaecomastia. New Engl J Med 1993; 328: 490.

Dixon JM, Mansel RE. Congenital problems and aberrations of normal development and involution. Br Med J 1994; 309: 797–800.

Jeffreys DB. Painful gynaecomastia treated with tamoxifen. Br Med J 1979; 1: 1119–1120.

Jones DJ, Davison DJ, Holt SD et al. A comparison of danazol and placebo in the treatment of adult idiopathic gynaecomastia: results of a prospective study in 55 patients. Ann Roy Coll Surg Engl 1990; 72: 296.

McDermott MT, Hofeldt FD, Kidd GS. Tamoxifen therapy for painful idiopathic gynaecomastia. South Med J 1990; 83: 1283.

Parker LN, Gray DR, Lai MK, Levin ER. Treatment of gynaecomastia with tamoxifen: a double-blind crossover study. Metabolism 1986; 35: 705–708.

Schnitt SJ, Connolly JL. Benign disorders. In: Diseases of the Breast. Eds: Harris JR, Lippman ME, Morrow M, Hellman S. Lippincott-Raven, Philadelphia, 1996, pp 27–41.

Breast pain

Cyclical breast pain

Boyd NF, Cousins M, McGuire V, Lockwood G, Tritchler D. Dietary intervention trials in subjects with benign breast disease. In: Recent Developments in the Study of Benign Breast Disease: The Proceedings of the 4th International Benign Breast Symposium. Ed.: Mansel RE. Parthenon Publishing Group, England, 1992, pp 59–74.

Fentiman IS, Caleffi M, Brame K, Chaudary MA, Hayward JL. Double blind controlled trial of tamoxifen therapy for mastalgia. Lancet 1986; i: 287–288.

Fentiman IS, Hamed H, Caleffi M. Experience with tamoxifen and goserelin in women with mastalgia. In: Recent Developments in the Study of Benign Breast Disease: The Proceedings of the 4th International Benign Breast Symposium. Ed.: Mansel RE. Parthenon Publishing Group, England, 1992, pp 23–26.

Gateley CA, Miers M, Mansel RE. The Cardiff mastalgia clinic experience of the drug treatments for mastalgia. In: Recent Developments in the Study of Benign Breast Disease: The Proceedings of the 4th International Benign Breast Symposium. Ed.: Mansel RE. Parthenon Publishing Group, England, 1992, pp 53–58.

Gateley CA, Miers M, Skone JF, Mansel RE. The Cardiff mastalgia clinic experience of the natural history of mastalgia. In: Recent Developments in the Study of Benign Breast Disease: The Proceedings of the 4th International Benign Breast Symposium. Ed.: Mansel RE. Parthenon Publishing Group, England, 1992, pp 17–22.

Hughes LE, Mansel RE, Webster DJT. Breast pain and nodularity. In: Benign Disorders and Diseases of the Breast: Concepts and Clinical Management. Bailliere Tindall, London, 1989, pp 75–92.

Kumar S, Mansel RE, Hughes LE, Woodhead JS, Edwards CA, Scanlon MF, Newcombe RG. Prolactin response to thyrotropin-releasing hormone stimulation and dopaminergic inhibition in benign breast disease. Cancer 1984; 53: 1311–1315.

Mansel RE. ABC of Breast Diseases: Breast Pain. Br Med J 1994; 309: 866–868.

Mansel RE, Wisbey JR, Hughes LE. Controlled trial of the antigonadotrophin danazol in painful nodular benign breast disease. Lancet 1982; i: 982–031.

Minton JP, Abou-Issa H, Reiches N, Roseman JM. Clinical and biochemical studies in methylxanthine-related fibrocystic breast disease. Surgery 1981; 90: 299–304.

Preece PE, Baum M, Mansel RE et al. The importance of mastalgia in operable breast cancer. Br Med J 1982; 284: 1299–1300.

Preece PE, Hughes LE, Mansel RE, Baum M, Bolton PM, Gravelle IH. Clinical syndromes of mastalgia. Lancet 1976; ii: 670–673.

Non-cyclical breast pain

Galea MH, Blamey RW. Non-cyclical breast pain: 1 year audit of an improved classification. In: Recent Developments in the Study of Benign Breast Disease: The Proceedings of the 4th International Benign Breast Symposium. Ed.: Mansel RE. Parthenon Publishing Group, England, 1992, pp 75–80.

Maddox PR, Harrison BJ, Mansel RE, Hughes LE. Non-cyclical mastalgia: an improved classification and treatment. Br J Surg 1989; 76: 901–904.

Pye JK, Mansel RE, Hughes LE. Clinical experience of drug treatment for mastalgia. Lancet 1985; i: 373–377.

Tietze A. A peculiar accumulation of cases with dystrophy of the cartilages of the ribs. Berl Klin Wochenschrift 1921; 30: 829–831.

Breast infection

Breast infection – lactating breast abscess

Dixon JM. Repeated aspiration of breast abscesses in lactating women. Br Med J 1988; 297: 1517–1518.

Dixon JM. Breast surgery. In: Infection in Surgical Practice. Ed.: Taylor EW. Oxford University Press, Oxford, 1992, pp 187–196.

Dixon JM. ABC of breast diseases: breast infection. Br Med J 1994; 309: 946–949.

Non-lactating infection/mammary duct fistula

Atkins HJB. Mammillary fistula. Br Med J 1955; 2: 1473–1474.

Bundred NJ. The aetiology of periductal mastitis. The Breast 1993; 2: 1-2.

Bundred NJ, Dixon JM, Lumsden AB, Radford D, Hood J, Miles RS, Chetty U, Forrest APM. Are the lesions of duct ectasia sterile? Br J Surg 1985; 72: 844-845.

Dixon JM. ABC of breast diseases: breast infection. Br Med J 1994; 309: 946-949.

Dixon JM, RaviSekar O, Chetty U, Anderson TJ. Periductal mastitis and duct ectasia: different conditions with different aetiologies. Br J Surg 1996; 83: 820-822.

Dixon JM, Thompson AM. Effective surgical treatment for mammillary fistula. Br J Surg 1991; 78: 1185-1186.

Haagensen CD. Mammary duct ectasia: a disease that may simulate cancer. Cancer 1951; 4: 749-761.

Hadfield GJ. Excision of the major duct system for benign disease of the breast. Br J Surg 1960; 47: 472-477.

Hughes LE, Mansel RE, Webster DJT. The duct ectasia/periductal mastitis complex. In: Benign Disorders and Diseases of the Breast: Concepts and Clinical Management. Bailliere Tindall, London, 1989, pp 107-131.

Leach RD, Eykyn SJ, Phillips I, Corrin B. Anaerobic subareolar breast abscess. Lancet 1979; i: 35-37.

Sandison AT, Walker JC. Inflammatory mastitis, mammary duct ectasia and mammillary fistula. Br J Surg 1962; 50: 57-64.

Peripheral breast infection

Dixon JM. ABC of breast diseases: breast infection. Br Med J 1994; 309: 946-949.

Scholefield JJ, Duncan JL, Rodgers K. Review of a hospital experience of breast abscesses. Br J Surg 1987; 74: 469.

Hidradenitis suppurativa

Harris BJ, Mudge M, Hughes LE. Recurrence after surgical treatment of hidradenitis suppurativa. Br Med J 1987; 294: 487-489.

Hughes LE, Mansel RE, Webster DJT. Miscellaneous conditions. In: Benign Disorders and Diseases of the Breast: Current Concepts and Clinical Management. Bailliere Tindall, London, 1989, pp 175-185.

Breast lumps

Breast lumps – fibroadenoma

Dent DM, Cant PF. Fibroadenoma. World J Surg 1989; 13: 706.

Dixon JM. Cystic disease and fibroadenoma of the breast: natural history and relation to breast cancer risk. In: Breast Disease: New Approaches. Eds: Stewart HJ, Anderson TJ, Forrest APM. Br Med Bull 1991; 47: 258-271.

Dixon JM. Techniques of and indications for breast biopsy. Curr Pract Surg 1993; 5: 142-148.

Dixon JM, Dobie V, Lamb J, Walsh JS, Chetty U. Assessment of the acceptability of conservative management of fibroadenoma of the breast. Br J Surg 1996; 83: 264-265.

DuPont WD, Page DL, Parl FF et al. Long-term risk of breast cancer in women with fibroadenoma. New Engl J Med 1994; 331: 10.

Houlihan MJ. Fibroadenoma and hamartoma. In: Diseases of the Breast: Eds: Harris JR, Lippman ME, Morrow M, Hellman S. Lippincott Raven, Philadelphia, 1996, pp 45-48.

Hughes LE, Mansel RE, Webster DJT. Aberrations of normal development and involution (ANDI): a new perspective on pathogenesis and nomenclature of benign breast disorders. Lancet 1987; ii: 1316-1319.

Hughes LE, Mansel RE, Webster DJT. Fibroadenoma and related tumours. In: Benign Disorders and Diseases of the Breast: Current Concepts and Clinical Management. Bailliere Tindall, London, 1989, pp 59-74.

Parks A. The microanatomy of the breast. Ann Roy Coll Surg Engl 1959; 25: 235-251.

Phyllodes tumours

Cosmacini P, Zurrida S, Veronesi P et al. Phyllodes tumor of the breast: mammographic experience in 99 cases. Eur J Radiology 1992; 15: 11.

Hines JR, Murad TM, Beal JM. Prognostic indicators in cytosarcoma phyllodes. Am J Surg 1987; 153: 276.

Norris HJ, Taylor HB. Relationship of histologic features to behaviour of cytosarcoma phyllodes: analysis of ninety-four cases. Cancer 1967; 20: 2090.

Palmer ML, De Risi DC, Pelikan A et al. Treatment options and recurrence potential for cytosarcoma phyllodes. Surg Gynecol Obstet 1990; 170: 193.

Petrek JA. Phyllodes tumours. In: Diseases of the Breast: Eds: Harris JR, Lippman ME, Morrow M, Hellman S. Lippincott Raven, Philadelphia, 1996, pp 863-869.

Salvadori B, Cusumano F, Del Bo R. et al. Surgical treatment of phyllodes tumors of breast. Cancer 1989; 63: 2532.

Breast cysts

Bruzzi P, Dogliotti L, Naldoni C, Bucchi L, Costantini M, Cicognani A, Torta M, Buzzie GF, Angeli A. Cohort study of association of risk of breast cancer with cyst type in women with gross cystic disease of the breast. Br Med J 1997; 314: 925-928.

Bundred NJ, West RR, O'Dowd J, Mansel RE. Is there an increased risk of breast cancer in women who have had a breast cyst aspirated? Br J Cancer 1991; 64: 953-955.

Chardot C, Varroyi A, Parach RM. Mastose fibro-kystique et cancer. Bull Cancer 1970; 57: 251-268.

Ciatto S, Biggeri A, Del Turco MR, Bartoli D, Iossa A. Risk of breast cancer subsequent to proven breast cystic disease. Eur J Cancer 1990; 26: 555-557.

Dixon JM. Common surgical ailments. Curr Pract Surg 1995; 7: 118-122.

Dixon JM. Cystic disease of the breast. In: Benign Breast Disease. Eds: Smallwood JA, Taylor I. Edward Arnold, London, 1990, pp 66-84.

Dixon JM, McDonald C, Elton RA, Miller WR. Risk of breast cancer in women with palpable breast cysts. New Engl J Med 1998 (in press).

Dixon JM, Lumsden AB, Miller WR. The relationship of cyst type to risk factors for breast cancer and subsequent development of breast cancer. Eur J Cancer Clin Oncol 1985; 21: 1047-1050.

Haagensen CD. Diseases of the Breast. 2nd ed. Philadelphia, WB Saunders 1971.

Haagensen CD, Bodian C, Haagensen DE. Breast Carcinoma Risk and Detection. Philadelphia, WB Saunders, 1981.

Harrington LE, Lesnick G. The association between gross cysts of the breast and breast cancer. Breast 1981; 7: 113-117.

Roberts MM, Jones V, Elton RA et al. Risk of breast cancer in women with a history of benign disease of the breast. Br Med J 1984; 288: 275-278.

Nipple problems

Nipple problems – bloodstained nipple discharge/discharge from nipple/areola

Chetty U. Nipple discharge. In: Benign Breast Disease. Eds: Smallwood JA, Taylor I. Edward Arnold, London, 1990, pp 85-95.

Dixon JM. Mansel RE. ABC of Breast Diseases: Symptoms, assessment and guidelines for referral. Br Med J 1994; 309: 722–726.

Hadfield GJ. Further experience of the operation for excision in the major duct system of the breast. Br J Surg 1968; 55: 530–535.

Hughes LE, Mansel RE, Webster DJT. Nipple discharge. In: Benign Disorders and Diseases of the Breast. Bailliere Tindall, London, 1989, pp 133–142.

Selzer MH, Perloff LJ, Kelley RI, Fitts WJ. The significance of age in patients with nipple discharge. Surg Gynecol Obstet 1970; 131: 519–522.

Recent-onset nipple inversion/retraction

Devitt JE. Benign breast disease in the postmenopausal woman. World J Surg 1989; 13: 731.

Dixon JM. Periductal mastitis/duct ectasia. World J Surg 1989; 13: 715.

Hughes LE, Mansel RE, Webster DJT. Disorders of the Nipple and Areola. In: Benign Disorders and Diseases of the Breast: Concepts and Clinical Management. Bailliere Tindall, London, 1989, pp 151–158.

Thomas WG, Williamson RCN, Davies JC et al. The clinical syndrome of mammary duct ectasia. Br J Surg 1982; 69: 423.

Walker JC, Sandison AT. Mammary duct ectasia: a clinical study. Br J Surg 1964; 51: 350.

Breast cancer

Increased risk of breast cancer due to family history

Austoker J. Screening for breast cancer: psychosocial issues. Oncology 1995; 23: 438–440.

Bilimoria M, Morrow M. The woman at increased risk for breast cancer: evaluation and management strategies. Ca Cancer J Clin 1995; 45: 263–278.

Black DM. The genetics of breast cancer. Eur J Cancer 1994; 30a: 1957–1961.

Bruzzi P. Tamoxifen for the prevention of breast cancer. Br Med J 1998: 316: 1181–1182.

Decker D. Prophylactic mastectomy for familial breast cancer. JAMA 1993; 269: 2608–2609.

Easton DF. The inherited component of cancer. Br Med Bull 1994; 50: 527–535.

Futreal PA, Liu Q, Shattuck-Eidens D et al. BRCA1 mutations in primary breast and ovarian carcinomas. Science 1994; 266: 120–122.

Hill ADK, Doyle JM, McDermott EW, O'Higgins NJ. Hereditary breast cancer. Br J Surg 1997; 84: 1334–1339.

Hoskins KF, Stopfer JE, Calzone KE et al. Assessment and counselling for women with a family history of breast cancer: a guide for clinicians. JAMA 1995; 273: 577–585.

Lynch HT, Watson P, Conway TA, Lynch JF. Natural history and age of onset of hereditary breast cancer. Cancer 1992; 69: 1404–1407.

Marcus JN, Watson P, Page DL. Hereditary breast cancer: pathobiology, prognosis and BRCA1 and BRCA2 gene linkage. Cancer 1996; 77: 697–709.

Morrow M. Identification and management of women at increased risk of breast cancer development. Breast Cancer Res Treat 1994; 31: 53–60.

Increased risk of invasive breast cancer due to atypical hyperplasia/ductal carcinoma *in situ*

Azzopardi J. Problems in Breast Pathology. Saunders, Philadelphia, 1979, pp 113–128.

Dupont WD. Converting relative risks to absolute risks: a geographical approach. Stat Med 1989; 8: 641–651.

Dupont WD, Page DL. Risk factors for breast cancer in women with proliferative breast disease. New Engl J Med 1985; 312: 146–151.

Dupont W, Page D, Rogers L, Pare F. Influence of exogenous estrogens, proliferative breast disease and other variables on breast cancer risk. Cancer 1989; 63: 948–957.

Morrow M, Schnitt SJ, Harris JR. Ductal carcinoma in situ. In: Diseases of the Breast. Eds: Harris JR, Lippman ME, Morrow M, Hellman S. Lippincott-Raven, Philadelphia, 1996, pp 355–368.

Page DL. The clinical significance of mammary epithelial hyperplasia. The Breast 1992; 1: 3–7.

Page DL, Dupont WD, Rogers LW, Rados MS. Atypical hyperplastic lesions of the female breast: a long-term follow-up study. Cancer 1985; 55: 2698–2708.

Premenopausal patient with a small operable breast cancer

Bonadonna G. Evolving concepts in systemic adjuvant treatment of breast cancer. Cancer Res 1992; 52: 2127.

Bonadonna G, Brusamolino E, Valagussa P et al. Combination chemotherapy as an adjuvant treatment in operable breast cancer. New Engl J Med 1976; 294: 405.

Bonadonna G, Valagussa P. Dose-response effect of adjuvant chemotherapy in breast cancer. New Engl J Med 1981; 304: 10.

Bostwick J, III. Aesthetic and Reconstructive Breast Surgery. Mosby, St Louis, 1983.

Bostwick J, III. Plastic and Reconstructive Breast Surgery. Quality Medical Publishing, Inc. St Louis, 1990.

Bundred NJ, Morgan DAL, Dixon JM. ABC of Breast Diseases: Management of regional nodes in breast cancer. Br Med J 1994; 309: 1222-1225.

Clark GM. Prognostic and predictive factors. In: Diseases of the Breast. Eds: Harris JR, Lippman ME, Morrow M, Hellman S. Lippincott-Raven, Philadelphia, 1996, pp 461-486.

Dixon JM. Breast conservation surgery. Recent Adv Surg 1993; 16: 43-61.

Dixon JM. Breast reconstruction after mastectomy. Br J Surg 1995; 82: 865-866.

Early Breast Cancer Trialists' Collaborative Group. Systemic treatment of early breast cancer by hormonal, cytotoxic or immune therapy. Lancet 1992; 339: 1, 71.

Early Breast Cancer Trialists' Collaborative Group. Ovarian ablation in early breast cancer: overview of the randomised trials. Lancet 1996; 348: 1189-1196.

Early Breast Cancer Trialists' Collaborative Group. Tamoxifen for early breast cancer: an overview of the randomised trials. Lancet 1998; 351: 1451-1467.

Fallowfield LJ, Hall A. Psychosocial and sexual impact of diagnosis and treatment of breast cancer. Br Med Bull 1991; 47: 388-399.

Fisher B, Anderson S, Redmond CK, Wolmark N, Wickerham DL, Cronin WM. Reanalysis and results after 12 years of follow-up in a randomized clinical trial comparing total mastectomy with lumpectomy with or without irradiation in the treatment of breast cancer. New Engl J Med 1995; 333: 1456-1461.

Foster RS. Techniques for the diagnosis of palpable breast masses. In: Diseases of the Breast. Eds: Harris JR, Lippman ME, Morrow M, Hellman S. Lippincott-Raven, Philadelphia 1996, pp 133-138.

Galimberti V, Zurrida S, Zucali P, Luini A. Can sentinel node biopsy avoid axillary dissection in clinically node-negative breast cancer patients? The Breast 1998; 7: 8-10.

Giuliano AE, Fitgan DM, Guenther JM, Morton DL. Lymphatic mapping and sentinel lymphadenectomy for breast cancer. Ann Surg 1994; 220: 391-401.

Goldhirsch A, Gelbert R. Adjuvant treatment for early breast cancer: the Ludwig breast cancer studies. Nat Cancer Inst Monogr 1986; 1: 55.

Goldwyn RM. Breast reconstruction after mastectomy. New Engl J Med 1987; 317: 1711.

Harris JR, Morrow M. Local management of invasive breast cancer. In: Diseases of the Breast. Eds: Harris JR, Lippman ME, Morrow M, Hellman S. Lippincott-Raven, Philadelphia, 1996, pp 487–547.

Hartrampf CR Jr. The transverse abdominal island flap for breast reconstruction. Clin Plast Surg 1988; 15: 703.

Lemperle G, Nievergelt J. Plastic and Reconstructive Breast Surgery: An Atlas. Springer-Verlag, Berlin, 1991.

McCraw JB, Horton CE, Grossman JA et al. An early appraisal of the methods of tissue expansion and the transverse rectus abdominis musculocutaneous flap in reconstruction of the breast following mastectomy. Ann Plast Surg 1987; 18: 93.

McGuire WL, Clark GM. Prognostic factors and treatment decisions in axillary-node-negative breast cancer. N Engl J Med 1992; 326: 1756–1761.

NATO Steering Committee. Controlled trial of tamoxifen as a single adjuvant agent in the management of early breast cancer. Br J Cancer 1988; 57: 608.

Osborne CK, Clark GM, Ravdin PM. Adjuvant systemic therapy of primary breast cancer. In: Diseases of the Breast. Eds: Harris JR, Lippman ME, Morrow M, Hellman S. Lippincott-Raven, Philadelphia, 1996, pp 548–578.

Recht A, Come SE, Henderson IC, Gelman RS et al. The sequencing of chemotherapy and radiation therapy after conservative surgery for early stage breast cancer. N Engl J Med 1996; 34: 1356–1361.

Report from the Breast Cancer Trials Committee, Scottish Cancer Trials Office, Edinburgh. Adjuvant tamoxifen in the management of operable breast cancer: the Scottish trial. Lancet 1987: 8552.

Sainsbury JRC, Anderson TJ, Morgan DAL, Dixon JM. Breast cancer. ABC of breast diseases: Breast cancer. Br Med J 1994; 309: 1150–1153.

Scottish Cancer Trials Breast Group and ICRF Breast Unit, Guy's Hospital. Adjuvant ovarian ablation versus CMF chemotherapy in premenopausal women with pathological stage II breast carcinoma: the Scottish trial. Lancet 1993; 341: 1293.

Silen W, Matory WE, Love SM. Atlas of Techniques in Breast Surgery: An Atlas. Lippincott-Raven, Philadelphia, 1996.

van der Veen H, Hoekstra OS, Paul MA, Cuesta MA, Meijer S. Gamma probe-guided sentinel node biopsy to select patients with melanoma for lymphadenectomy. Br J Surg 1994; 81: 1769–1770.

Veronesi U, Banfi A, Salvadori B et al. Breast conservation is the treatment of choice in small breast cancer: long-term results of a randomized clinical trial. Eur J Cancer 1990; 26: 668.

Veronesi U, Volterrani F, Luini A et al. Quadrantectomy versus lumpectomy for small size breast cancer. Eur J Cancer 1990; 26: 671.

Watson JD, Sainsbury JRC, Dixon JM. ABC of Breast Diseases: Breast reconstruction after surgery. Br Med J 1995; 310: 117–121.

Webster DJT, Mansel RE, Hughes LE. Immediate reconstruction of the breast after mastectomy: is it safe? Cancer 1984; 53: 1416.

Winchester D, Cox J. Standards for breast conservation treatment. Ca Cancer J Clin 1992; 42: 134–144.

Young VL, Lund H, Ueda K, Pidgeon L, Watson Schorr M, Kreeger J. Bleed of and biologic response to triglyceride filler used in radiolucent breast implants. Plast Reconstr Surg 1996; 97: 1179–1193.

Premenopausal patient with a small operable breast cancer

Bonadonna G. Evolving concepts in systemic adjuvant treatment of breast cancer. Cancer Res 1992; 52: 2127.

Bonadonna G, Brusamolino E, Valagussa P et al. Combination chemotherapy as an adjuvant treatment in operable breast cancer. New Engl J Med 1976; 294: 405.

Bonadonna G, Valagussa P. Dose-response effect of adjuvant chemotherapy in breast cancer. New Engl J Med 1981; 304: 10.

Bonadonna G, Valgussa P, Brambilla C et al. Adjuvant and neoadjuvant treatment of breast cancer with chemotherapy and/or endocrine therapy. Semin Oncol 1991; 51: 515–524.

Bostwick J, III. Aesthetic and Reconstructive Breast Surgery. Mosby, St Louis, 1983.

Bostwick J, III. Plastic and Reconstructive Breast Surgery. Quality Medical Publishing, Inc. St Louis, 1990.

Bundred NJ, Morgan DAL, Dixon JM. ABC of Breast Diseases: Management of regional nodes in breast cancer. Br Med J 1994; 309: 1222–1225.

Clark GM. Prognostic and predictive factors. In: Diseases of the Breast. Eds: Harris JR, Lippman ME, Morrow M, Hellman S. Lippincott-Raven, Philadelphia, 1996, pp 461–486.

Dixon JM. Breast conservation surgery. Recent Adv Surg 1993; 16: 43–61.

Dixon JM. Breast reconstruction after mastectomy. Br J Surg 1995; 82: 865–866.

Early Breast Cancer Trialists' Collaborative Group. Systemic treatment of early breast cancer by hormonal, cytotoxic or immune therapy. Lancet 1992; 339: 1, 71.

Early Breast Cancer Trialists' Collaborative Group. Ovarian ablation in early breast cancer: overview of the randomised trials. Lancet 1996; 348: 1189–1196.

Early Breast Cancer Trialists' Collaborative Group. Tamoxifen for early breast cancer: an overview of the randomised trials. Lancet 1998; 351: 1451–1467.

Fallowfield LJ, Hall A. Psychosocial and sexual impact of diagnosis and treatment of breast cancer. Br Med Bull 1991; 47: 388–399.

Fisher B, Anderson S, Redmond CK, Wolmark N, Wickerham DL, Cronin WM. Reanalysis and results after 12 years of follow-up in a randomized clinical trial comparing total mastectomy with lumpectomy with or without irradiation in the treatment of breast cancer. New Engl J Med 1995; 333: 1456–1461.

Fisher B, Brown A, Mamounis E et al. Effect of pre-operative chemotherapy on local regional disease on women with operable breast cancer: findings from National Surgical Adjuvant Breast and Bowel Project N18. J Clin Oncol 1997; 15: 2483–2493.

Foster RS. Techniques for the diagnosis of palpable breast masses. In: Diseases of the Breast. Eds: Harris JR, Lippman ME, Morrow M, Hellman S. Lippincott-Raven, Philadelphia, 1996, pp 133–138.

Galimberti V, Zurrida S, Zucali P, Luini A. Can sentinel node biopsy avoid axillary dissection in clinically node-negative breast cancer patients? The Breast 1998; 7: 8–10.

Giuliano AE, Fitgan DM, Guenther JM, Morton DL. Lymphatic mapping and sentinel lymphadenectomy for breast cancer. Ann Surg 1994; 220: 391–401.

Goldhirsch A, Gelbert R. Adjuvant treatment for early breast cancer: the Ludwig breast cancer studies. Nat Cancer Inst Monogr 1986; 1: 55.

Goldwyn RM. Breast reconstruction after mastectomy. New Engl J Med 1987; 317: 1711.

Harris JR, Morrow M. Local management of invasive breast cancer. In: Diseases of the Breast. Eds: Harris JR, Lippman ME, Morrow M, Hellman S. Lippincott-Raven, Philadelphia, 1996, pp 487–547.

Hartrampf CR Jr. The transverse abdominal island flap for breast reconstruction. Clin Plast Surg 1988; 15: 703.

Lemperle G, Nievergelt J. Plastic and Reconstructive Breast Surgery: An Atlas. Springer-Verlag, Berlin, 1991.

McCraw JB, Horton CE, Grossman JA et al. An early appraisal of the methods of tissue expansion and the transverse rectus abdominis musculocutaneous flap in reconstruction of the breast following mastectomy. Ann Plast Surg 1987; 18: 93.

McGuire WL, Clark GM. Prognostic factors and treatment decisions in axillary-node-negative breast cancer. N Engl J Med 1992; 326: 1756–1761.

Mauriac L, Durand M, Avril A et al. Effects of primary chemotherapy in conservative treatment of breast cancer patients with operable tumours larger than 3 cm: results of a randomised trial in a single centre. Ann Oncol 1991; 2: 347–354.

NATO Steering Committee. Controlled trial of tamoxifen as a single adjuvant agent in the management of early breast cancer. Br J Cancer 1988; 57: 608.

Osborne CK, Clark GM, Ravdin PM. Adjuvant systemic therapy of primary breast cancer. In: Diseases of the Breast. Eds: Harris JR, Lippman ME, Morrow M, Hellman S. Lippincott-Raven, Philadelphia, 1996, pp 548–578.

Recht A, Come SE, Henderson IC, Gelman RS et al. The sequencing of chemotherapy and radiation therapy after conservative surgery for early stage breast cancer. N Engl J Med 1996; 34: 1356–1361.

Report from the Breast Cancer Trials Committee, Scottish Cancer Trials Office, Edinburgh. Adjuvant tamoxifen in the management of operable breast cancer: the Scottish trial. Lancet 1987: 8552.

Sainsbury JRC, Anderson TJ, Morgan DAL, Dixon JM. Breast cancer. ABC of breast diseases: Breast cancer. Br Med J 1994; 309: 1150–1153.

Scottish Cancer Trials Breast Group and ICRF Breast Unit, Guy's Hospital. Adjuvant ovarian ablation versus CMF chemotherapy in premenopausal women with pathological stage II breast carcinoma: the Scottish trial. Lancet 1993; 341: 1293.

Silen W, Matory WE, Love SM. Atlas of Techniques in Breast Surgery: An Atlas. Lippincott-Raven, Philadelphia, 1996.

Smith IE. Primary (neoadjuvant) medical therapy: introduction. In: Medical Management of Breast Cancer. Eds: Powles T, Smith IE. London, Martin-Dunitz, 1991, pp 259–265.

van der Veen H, Hoekstra OS, Paul MA, Cuesta MA, Meijer S. Gamma probe-guided sentinel node biopsy to select patients with melanoma for lymphadenectomy. Br J Surg 1994; 81: 1769–1770.

Veronesi U, Banfi A, Salvadori B et al. Breast conservation is the treatment of choice in small breast cancer: long-term results of a randomized clinical trial. Eur J Cancer 1990; 26: 668.

Veronesi U, Volterrani F, Luini A et al. Quadrantectomy versus lumpectomy for small size breast cancer. Eur J Cancer 1990; 26: 671.

Watson JD, Sainsbury JRC, Dixon JM. ABC of Breast Diseases: Breast reconstruction after surgery. Br Med J 1995; 310: 117-121.

Webster DJT, Mansel RE, Hughes LE. Immediate reconstruction of the breast after mastectomy: is it safe? Cancer 1984; 53: 1416.

Winchester D, Cox J. Standards for breast conservation treatment. Ca Cancer J Clin 1992; 42: 134-144.

Young VL, Lund H, Ueda K, Pidgeon L, Watson Schorr M, Kreeger J. Bleed of and biologic response to triglyceride filler used in radiolucent breast implants. Plast Reconstr Surg 1996; 97: 1179-1193.

Post-menopausal patient with large operable breast cancer

Anderson EDC, Forrest APM, Levack PA et al. Response to endocrine manipulation in large, operable breast cancer. Br J Cancer 1989; 60: 223-260.

Becker H. The permanent tissue expander. Clin Plast Surg 1987; 14: 519.

Bonadonna G, Valgussa P, Brambilla C et al. Adjuvant and neoadjuvant treatment of breast cancer with chemotherapy and/or endocrine therapy. Semin Oncol 1991; 15: 515-524.

Bundred NJ, Morgan DAL, Dixon JM. ABC of Breast Diseases: Management of regional nodes in breast cancer. Br Med J 1994; 309: 1222-1225.

Dixon JM. ABC of Breast Diseases. BMJ Publishing Group, London, 1995.

Dixon JM, Leonard RCF. Hormones and chemotherapy. In: Breast and Endocrine Surgery: A Companion to Specialist Surgical Practice. Ed.: Farndon JR. WB Saunders, London, 1997, pp 275-308.

Early Breast Cancer Trialists' Collaborative Group. Systemic treatment of early breast cancer by hormonal, cytotoxic, or immune therapy. 133 randomised trials involving 3100 recurrence and 24000 deaths among 75000 women. Lancet 1992; 339: 1-15, 71-85.

Early Breast Cancer Trialists' Collaborative Group. Tamoxifen for early breast cancer: an overview of the randomised trials. Lancet 1998; 351: 1451-1467.

Forrest APM, Anderson EDC, Gaskill D. Primary systemic therapy. In: Breast Cancer: New Approaches. Eds: Stewart HJ, Anderson TJ, Forrest APM. Br Med Bull 1991; 47: 357-371.

Gibney J. The long term results of tissue expansion for breast reconstruction. Clin Plast Surg 1987; 14: 509.

Goldhirsch A, Wood WC, Senn HJ, Glick JH et al. Meeting highlights: International consensus panel on the treatment of primary breast cancer. J Natl Cancer Inst 1995; 87: 1441-1445.

Gruber RP, Khan RA, Lash H et al. Breast reconstruction following mastectomy: a comparison of submuscular and subcutaneous techniques. Plast Reconstr Surg 1981; 67: 312.

Gylbert L, Asplung O, Jurell G. Capsular contracture after breast reconstruction with silicone-gel and saline-filled implants: a 6 year follow up. Plast Reconstr Surg 1990; 85: 373.

Hortobagyi GN, Singletary SE, McNeese MD. Treatment of locally advanced and inflammatory breast cancer. In: Diseases of the Breast. Eds: Harris JR, Lippman ME, Morrow M, Hellman S. Lippincott-Raven, Philadelphia, 1996, pp 585–599.

Loprinzi CL, Michalak JC, Quella SK. Megestrol acetate for the prevention of hot flashes. New Engl J Med 1994; 331: 347–352.

Mauriac L, Durand M, Avril M et al. Effects of primary chemotherapy in conservative treatment of breast cancer patients with operable tumours larger than 3 cm: results of a randomised trial in a single centre. Ann Oncol 1991; 2: 347–354.

Nemoto T, Vana J, Bedwani RN, Baker HW et al. Management and survival of female breast cancer: results of national survey by the American College of Surgeons. Cancer 1980; 45: 2917–2924.

Radovan C. Breast reconstruction after mastectomy using a temporary expander. Plast Reconstr Surg 1982; 69: 195.

Sainsbury JRC, Anderson TJ, Morgan DAL, Dixon JM. Breast cancer. ABC of breast diseases: breast cancer. Br Med J 1994; 309: 1150–1153.

Smith IE. Primary (neoadjuvant) medical therapy: introduction. In: Medical Management of Breast Cancer. Eds: Powles T, Smith IE. Martin-Dunitz, London, 1991, pp 259–265.

Smith IE, Walsh G, Jones A et al. High complete remission rate with primary neoadjuvant infusional chemotherapy for large early breast cancer. J Clin Oncol 1995; 13: 424–429.

A screen-detected mass in a post-menopausal woman

Chave MJB, Flowers CI, O'Brien CJ et al. Image-guided core biopsy in patients with breast disease. Br J Surg 1996; 83: 1415–1416.

Kertilowske K, Grady D, Rubin S et al. Efficacy of screening mammography, a meta-analysis. JAMA 1995; 273: 149–154.

Kissin MW. Breast screening and screen-detected disease. In: Breast and Endocrine Surgery: A Companion to Specialist Surgical Practice. Ed.: Farndon JR. WB Saunders, London, 1997, pp 215–242.

Litherland JC, Evans AJ, Wilson ARM et al. The impact of core-biopsy on pre-operative diagnosis rate of screen detected breast cancers. Clin Radiol 1996; 51: 562–565.

Morrow M. Axillary dissection: when and how radical? Semin Surg Oncol 1996; 12: 321–327.

Morrow M, Harris JR, Schnitt SJ. Local control following breast-conserving surgery for invasive cancer: results of clinical trials. J Natl Cancer Inst 1995; 87: 1669–1673.

Nystrom L, Lutquist RLE, Wall S et al. Breast cancer screening with mammography over-view of Swedish randomised trials. Lancet 1993; 341: 973–978.

Sastre-Garau X, Jouce M, Asselain B et al. Infiltrating lobular carcinoma of the breast: clinicopathologic analysis of 975 cases with reference to data on conservative therapy and metastatic pattern. Cancer 1996; 77: 113–120.

Wald N, Murphy P, Major PE et al. UKCCCR multi-centre randomised control trial of one and two view mammography in breast cancer screening. Br Med J 1995; 311: 1189–1192.

Breast screening

Chave MJB, Flowers CI, O'Brien CJ et al. Image-guided core biopsy in patients with breast disease. Br J Surg 1996; 83: 1415–1416.

Kertilowske K, Grady D, Rubin S et al. Efficacy of screening mammography, a meta-analysis. JAMA 1995; 273: 149–154.

Kissin MW. Breast screening and screen-detected disease. In: Breast and Endocrine Surgery: A Companion to Specialist Surgical Practice. Ed.: Farndon JR. WB Saunders, London, 1997, pp 215–242.

Litherland JC, Evans AJ, Wilson ARM et al. The impact of core-biopsy on pre-operative diagnosis rate of screen detected breast cancers. Clin Radiol 1996; 51: 562–565.

Nystrom L, Lutquist RLE, Wall S et al. Breast cancer screening with mammography over-view of Swedish randomised trials. Lancet 1993; 341: 973–978.

Wald N, Murphy P, Major PE et al. UKCCCR multi-centre randomised control trial of one and two view mammography in breast cancer screening. Br Med J 1995; 311: 1189–1192.

Pre-menopausal patient with inflammatory breast cancer

Antman KH. Dose-intensive therapy in breast cancer. In: High-Dose Cancer Therapy. Eds: Armitage JO, Antman KH. Williams and Wilkins, Baltimore, 1992, pp 701.

deDycker RP, Timmerman J, Neumann RLA. Regional induction chemotherapy in locally advanced breast cancer. The Breast 1992; 1: 82–86.

De Lena M, Zucali R, Viganotti G, Valagussa P, Bonadonna G. Combined
chemotherapy-radiotherapy approach in locally advanced (T_{3b}-T_4) breast
cancer. Cancer Chemother Pharmacol 1978; 1: 53–59.

Harris JR, Sawicka J, Gleman R et al. Management of locally advanced
carcinoma of the breast by primary radiation therapy. Int J Radiat Oncol
Biol Physics 1983; 9: 345.

Hortobagyi GN, Singletary SE, McNeese MD. Treatment of locally advanced
and inflammatory breast cancer. In: Diseases of the Breast. Eds: Harris JR,
Lippman ME, Morrow M, Hellman S. Lippincott-Raven, Philadelphia, 1996,
pp 585–599.

Jaiyesimi IA, Buzdar AU, Hortobagyi G. Inflammatory breast cancer: a review.
J Clin Oncol 1992; 10: 1014.

Keiling R, Guiochet N, Calderoli H et al. Preoperative chemotherapy in the
treatment of inflammatory breast cancer. In: Primary Chemotherapy in
Cancer Medicine. Eds: Wagener DJT, Blijham GH, Smeets JBE et al. Alan R
Liss, New York, 1985, pp 95.

Zucali R, Islenghi C, Kenda R et al. Natural history and survival of inoperable
breast cancer treated with radiotherapy and radiotherapy followed by
radical mastectomy. Cancer 1976; 37: 1422.

Ulcerated locally advanced breast cancer

Hausheer FH, Yarbro JW. Diagnosis and treatment of malignant pleural
effusion. Semin Oncol 1985; 12: 54.

Pearson FG, Macgregor DC. Talc poudrage for malignant pleural effusion.
J Thoracic Cardiovasc Surg 1966; 51: 732.

Prakash UBS, Reiman HM. Comparison of needle biopsy with cytologic
analysis for the evaluation of pleural effusion: analysis of 414 cases. Mayo
Clinic Proc 1985; 60: 158.

Ruckdeschel JC, Moores D, Lee JY et al. Intrapleural therapy for malignant
pleural effusions: a randomised comparison of bleomycin and tetracycline.
Chest 1991; 100: 1528–1535.

Patient presenting with metastatic breast cancer

Aaron AD, Jennings LC, Springfield DS. Local treatment of bone metastases.
In: Diseases of the Breast. Eds: Harris JR, Lippman ME, Morrow M,
Hellman S. Lippincott-Raven, Philadelphia, 1996, pp 811–819.

Bezwoda WR, Seymour L, Dansey RD. High-dose chemotherapy with haematopoietic rescue as primary treatment for metastatic breast cancer: a randomized trial. J Clin Oncol 1995; 13: 2483–2489.

Bundred NJ, Morgan DAL, Dixon JM. ABC of Breast Diseases: Management of regional nodes in breast cancer. Br Med J 1994; 309: 1222–1225.

Come SE, Schnipper LE. Bone marrow metastases. In: Diseases of the Breast. Eds: Harris JR, Lippman ME, Morrow M, Hellman S. Lippincott-Raven, Philadelphia, 1996, pp 847–853.

Gradishar WJ, Tallman MS, Abrams JS. High-dose chemotherapy for breast cancer. Ann Int Med 1996; 125: 599–604.

Hausheer FH, Yabro JW. Diagnosis and treatment of malignant pleural effusion. Semin Oncol 1985; 12: 54.

Honig SF. Hormonal therapy and chemotherapy. In: Diseases of the Breast. Eds: Harris JR, Lippman ME, Morrow M, Hellman S. Lippincott-Raven, Philadelphia, 1996, pp 669–734.

Hortobagyi GN, Theriault RL, Porter L et al. Efficacy of pamidronate in reducing skeletal complications in patients with breast cancer and lytic bone metastases. New Engl J Med 1996; 355: 1785–1791.

Myers SE, Williams SF. Role of high-dose chemotherapy and autologous stem cell support in treatment of breast cancer. Hematol Oncol Clinics North Am 1993; 7: 631–645.

Robinson RG, Blake GM, Preston DF et al. Strontium-89: treatment results and kinetics in patients with painful metastatic prostate and breast cancer in bone. Radiography 1989; 9: 271.

Theriault RL. Medical treatment of bone metastases. In: Diseases of the Breast. Eds: Harris JR, Lippman ME, Morrow M, Hellman S. Lippincott-Raven, Philadelphia, 1996, pp 819–826.

Tannock IF, Boyd NF, DoBoer G et al. A randomized trial of two dose levels of cyclophosphamide, methetrexate and fluorouracil chemotherapy for patients with metastatic breast cancer. J Clin Oncol 1988; 6: 137.

Warrell RP Jr. Hypercalcaemia. In: Diseases of the Breast. Eds: Harris JR, Lippman ME, Morrow M, Hellman S. Lippincott-Raven, Philadelphia, 1996, pp 840–847.

Patient presenting with isolated axillary nodal metastasis

Baron PL, Moore MP, Kinne DW et al. Occult breast cancer presenting with axillary metastases: updated management. Arch Surg 1990; 125: 210.

Bundred NJ, Morgan DAL, Dixon JM. ABC of Breast Diseases: Management of regional nodes in breast cancer. Br Med J 1994; 309: 1222–1225.

Diel IJ, Solomayer EF, Costa S et al. Reduction in new metastases in breast cancer with adjuvant clodronate treatment. New Eng J Med 1998; 339: 357–400.

Fourquet A, de la Rochefordiere A, Campana F. Occult primary cancer with axillary metastases. In: Diseases of the Breast. Eds: Harris JR, Lippman ME, Morrow M, Hellman S. Lippincott Raven, Philadelphia, 1996, pp 892–896.

Local recurrence following mastectomy

Blacklay PF, Campbell FS, Hinton SP et al. Patterns of flap recurrence following mastectomy. Br J Surg 1995; 72: 917–920.

Ng JSY, Cameron DA, Lee L et al. Infusional 5-fluorouracil given as a single agent in relapsed breast cancer: its activity and toxicity. The Breast 1994; 2: 87–90.

Sainsbury JRC, Anderson TJ, Morgan DAL, Dixon JM. ABC of breast diseases: breast cancer. Br Med J 1994; 309: 1150–1153.

Valagussa P, Bonadonna G, Veronesi U. Patterns of relapse and survival following radical mastectomy. Cancer 1978; 41: 1170.

Male breast cancer

Black DM. The genetics of breast cancer. Eur J Cancer 1994; 30a: 1957–1961.

Easton DF. The inherited component of cancer. Br Med Bull 1994; 50: 527–535.

Hill ADK, Doyle JM, McDermott EW, O'Higgins NJ. Hereditary breast cancer. Br J Surg 1997; 84: 1334–1339.

Lynch HT, Watson P, Conway TA, Lynch JF. Natural history and age of onset of hereditary breast cancer. Cancer 1992; 69: 1404–1407.

Marcus JN, Watson P, Page DL. Hereditary breast cancer: pathobiology, prognosis and BRCA1 and BRCA2 gene linkage. Cancer 1996; 77: 697–709.

Moore MP. Male breast cancer. In: Diseases of the Breast. Eds: Harris JR, Lippman ME, Morrow M, Hellman S. Lippincott-Raven, Philadelphia, 1996, pp 859–862.

Levy-Lahad E, Catane R, Eisenberg S et al. Founder BRCA1 and BRCA2 mutations in Ashkenasi Jews in Israel: frequency and differential penetrance in ovarian cancer and breast-ovarian cancer families. Am J Human Genet 1997; 60: 1079–1084.

Memori MA, Donohue JH. Male breast cancer. Br J Surg 1997; 84: 433–435.

Ribeiro GG, Swindell R, Harris M, Banerjee SS, Cramer A. A review of the management of male breast cancer based on an analysis of 420 treated cases. The Breast 1996; 6: 141–146.

Thorlacius S, Olafsdottir G, Trygvadottir R et al. A single BRCA2 mutation in male and female breast cancer families from Iceland with varied cancer phenotypes. Nature Genet 1996; 13: 117–119.

Wooster R, Bignell G, Lancaster J et al. Identification of the breast cancer susceptibility gene BRCA2. Nature 1995; 378: 789–792.

Psychological problems

Fallowfield LJ, Hall A, Maguire GP, Baum M. Psychological outcomes of different treatment policies in women with early breast cancer outside a clinical trial. Br Med J 1990; 301: 575–580.

Greer S, Moorey S, Baruch JK et al. Adjuvant psychological therapy for patients with cancer: a prospective randomised trial. Br Med J 1992; 304: 675–680.

Harrison J, Maguire P. Predictors of psychiatric morbidity in cancer patients. Br J Psychiatry 1994; 165: 5933–5938.

Harrison J, Maguire P, Ibbotson T, MacLeod R, Hopwood P. Concerns, confiding and psychiatric disorder in newly diagnosed cancer patients: a descriptive study. Psycho-Oncol 1994; 3: 173–179.

Ibbotson T, Maguire P, Selby P. Priestman T, Wallace L. Screening for anxiety and depression in cancer patients: effects of disease and treatment. Eur J Cancer 1994; 30a: 37–40.

Maguire P. ABC of Breast Disease: psychological aspects. Br Med J 1994; 309: 1649–1652.

Maguire P. Improving the recognition and treatment of affective disorders in cancer patients. In: Recent Advances in Clinical Psychiatry. Ed.: Granville Grossman K. Churchill Livingstone, Edinburgh, 1992, pp 15–30.

Parle M, Jones B, Maguire P. Maladaptive coping and affective disorders in cancer patients. Psychol Med 1996; 26: 735–744.

Index

Note: page numbers in italics refer to figures and tables

implants *see* prostheses; silicone, implants; tissue expanders

infection

hidradenitis suppurativa 45, 46

peripheral 42-3

skin 45-6

intertrigo, submammary 11

involution 63, 70-1

iridium wire 115

Klinefelter syndrome 23, 25, 177

lactating infection 35-7

abscess 37-9

laminectomy, decompression 164

latissimus dorsi muscle flap 58, 60

breast reconstruction 111, 113

reconstruction 7, 91

tissue replacement in mastectomy 120

lentaron 173

letrozole 173

Li-Fraumeni syndrome 76

linguine sign *21*

liposuction 23

liver disease, metastatic 124-5, 126, 163-4

lobular carcinoma *in situ* 87

local recurrence 169

breast conservation 100-3, 109

time to relapse 110

locally advanced breast cancer (LABC) 153-4, 159-61

conservation therapy 156-7

neo-adjuvant chemotherapy 154, 155-6

oestrogen-positive 159

lorazepam 181

lumpectomy

axillary dissection 100-3

DCIS 110

infiltrating carcinoma 110

irradiation 103, 145

recurrence 103

lung metastases 60, 163-4